Patient Narcotic's Log

Häfliger 1917 - Switzerland

User Data Page

Book Number:

Subject:

Continued from book number: Continued to book number:

Issue / Start Date: End Date:

Issued to (name):

Signature: Date:

Issued by: Date:

Phone Number:

Email:

Company / Organization:

Department:

Street Address:

City: State: Zip:

Notes:

Patient Index

Page #	Patient Name	Drug Name / Rx #	Physician	Start Date	End Date
1					
2					
3					
4					
5					
6					
7					
8					
9					
10					
11					
12					
13					
14					
15					
16					
17					
18					
19					
20					
21					
22					
23					
24					
25					
26					
27					
28					
29					
30					
31					
32					
33					
34					
35					

Patient Index

Page #	Patient Name	Drug Name / Rx #	Physician	Start Date	End Date
36					
37					
38					
39					
40					
41					
42					
43					
44					
45					
46					
47					
48					
49					
50					
51					
52					
53					
54					
55					
56					
57					
58					
59					
60					
61					
62					
63					
64					
65					
66					
67					
68					
69					
70					

Patient Index

Page #	Patient Name	Drug Name / Rx #	Physician	Start Date	End Date
71					
72					
73					
74					
75					
76					
77					
78					
79					
80					
81					
82					
83					
84					
85					
86					
87					
88					
89					
90					
91					
92					
93					
94					
95					
96					
97					
98					
99					
100					
101					
102					
103					
104					
105					

Patient Index

Page #	Patient Name	Drug Name / Rx #	Physician	Start Date	End Date
106					
107					
108					
109					
110					
111					
112					
113					
114					
115					
116					
117					
118					
119					
120					
121					
122					
123					
124					
125					
126					
127					
128					
129					
130					

PATIENT NARCOTIC'S LOG

Page Start Date	From Page #	To Page #

Patient Information

Last Name	First Name	Middle Name/Init.	Room #	Bed#

Medication Name	Rx #	Prescribing Physician

☐ Oral	☐ Hypo	☐ Rectal	Initial Quantity Rec'd	Date Received	Pharmacy

Dosage / Directions

#	Date	Time	On Hand	Quantity Given	Quantity Rem-aining	From RX	Nurse Signature	Verified By Signature	Date	Time	Notes
1											
2											
3											
4											
5											
6											
7											
8											
9											
10											
11											
12											
13											
14											
15											
16											

Drug Depleted?	Date	Time	Signature

Date	Medication Quantity Remaining	Authorized Signature

Disposition of Unused Drug

Date	Disposition Method / Notes	Authorized Signature

PATIENT NARCOTIC'S LOG

Page Start Date	From Page #	To Page #

Patient Information

Last Name	First Name	Middle Name/Init.	Room #	Bed#

Medication Name	Rx #	Prescribing Physician

			Initial Quantity Rec'd	Date Received	Pharmacy
☐ Oral	☐ Hypo	☐ Rectal			

Dosage / Directions

#	Date	Time	Quantity On Hand	Quantity Given	Quantity Rem-aining	Quantity From RX	Nurse Signature	Verified By Signature	Date	Time	Notes
1											
2											
3											
4											
5											
6											
7											
8											
9											
10											
11											
12											
13											
14											
15											
16											

Drug Depleted?	Date	Time	Signature

Date	Medication Quantity Remaining	Authorized Signature

Disposition of Unused Drug

Date	Disposition Method / Notes	Authorized Signature

PATIENT NARCOTIC'S LOG

Page Start Date	From Page #	To Page #

Patient Information

Last Name	First Name	Middle Name/Init.	Room #	Bed#

Medication Name	Rx #	Prescribing Physician

☐ Oral	☐ Hypo	☐ Rectal	Initial Quantity Rec'd	Date Received	Pharmacy

Dosage / Directions

#	Date	Time	On Hand	Given	Rem-aining	From RX	Nurse Signature	Verified By Signature	Date	Time	Notes
1											
2											
3											
4											
5											
6											
7											
8											
9											
10											
11											
12											
13											
14											
15											
16											

(Quantity spans: On Hand, Given, Rem-aining, From RX)

Drug Depleted?	Date	Time	Signature

Date	Medication Quantity Remaining	Authorized Signature

Disposition of Unused Drug

Date	Disposition Method / Notes	Authorized Signature

PATIENT NARCOTIC'S LOG

Page Start Date	From Page #	To Page #

Patient Information

Last Name	First Name	Middle Name/Init.	Room #	Bed#

Medication Name	Rx #	Prescribing Physician

☐ Oral	☐ Hypo	☐ Rectal	Initial Quantity Rec'd	Date Received	Pharmacy

Dosage / Directions

#	Date	Time	On Hand	Quantity Given	Quantity Rem-aining	From RX	Nurse Signature	Verified By Signature	Date	Time	Notes
1											
2											
3											
4											
5											
6											
7											
8											
9											
10											
11											
12											
13											
14											
15											
16											

Drug Depleted?	Date	Time	Signature

Date	Medication Quantity Remaining	Authorized Signature

Disposition of Unused Drug

Date	Disposition Method / Notes	Authorized Signature

PATIENT NARCOTIC'S LOG

Page Start Date	From Page #	To Page #

Patient Information

Last Name	First Name	Middle Name/Init.	Room # Bed#

Medication Name	Rx #	Prescribing Physician

☐ Oral	☐ Hypo	☐ Rectal	Initial Quantity Rec'd	Date Received	Pharmacy

Dosage / Directions

#	Date	Time	On Hand	Quantity Given	Quantity Rem-aining	From RX	Nurse Signature	Verified By Signature	Date	Time	Notes
1											
2											
3											
4											
5											
6											
7											
8											
9											
10											
11											
12											
13											
14											
15											
16											

Drug Depleted?	Date	Time	Signature

Date	Medication Quantity Remaining	Authorized Signature

Disposition of Unused Drug

Date	Disposition Method / Notes	Authorized Signature

PATIENT NARCOTIC'S LOG

Page Start Date	From Page #	To Page #

Patient Information

Last Name	First Name	Middle Name/Init.	Room #	Bed#

Medication Name	Rx #	Prescribing Physician

☐ Oral	☐ Hypo	☐ Rectal	Initial Quantity Rec'd	Date Received	Pharmacy

Dosage / Directions

#	Date	Time	On Hand	Given	Remaining	From RX	Nurse Signature	Verified By Signature	Date	Time	Notes
1											
2											
3											
4											
5											
6											
7											
8											
9											
10											
11											
12											
13											
14											
15											
16											

Drug Depleted?	Date	Time	Signature

Date	Medication Quantity Remaining	Authorized Signature

Disposition of Unused Drug

Date	Disposition Method / Notes	Authorized Signature

PATIENT NARCOTIC'S LOG

Page Start Date	From Page #	To Page #

Patient Information

Last Name	First Name	Middle Name/Init.	Room # Bed#

Medication Name	Rx #	Prescribing Physician

			Initial Quantity Rec'd	Date Received	Pharmacy
☐ Oral	☐ Hypo	☐ Rectal			

Dosage / Directions

#	Date	Time	On Hand	Given	Rem-aining	From RX	Nurse Signature	Verified By Signature	Date	Time	Notes
1											
2											
3											
4											
5											
6											
7											
8											
9											
10											
11											
12											
13											
14											
15											
16											

(Quantity spans On Hand, Given, Rem-aining, From RX columns)

Drug Depleted?	Date	Time	Signature

Date	Medication Quantity Remaining	Authorized Signature

Disposition of Unused Drug

Date	Disposition Method / Notes	Authorized Signature

PATIENT NARCOTIC'S LOG

	Page Start Date	From Page #	To Page #

Patient Information

Last Name	First Name	Middle Name/Init.	Room #	Bed#

Medication Name	Rx #	Prescribing Physician

☐	☐	☐	Initial Quantity Rec'd	Date Received	Pharmacy
Oral	Hypo	Rectal			

Dosage / Directions

#	Date	Time	Quantity On Hand	Given	Rem-aining	From RX	Nurse Signature	Verified By Signature	Date	Time	Notes
1											
2											
3											
4											
5											
6											
7											
8											
9											
10											
11											
12											
13											
14											
15											
16											

Drug Depleted?	Date	Time	Signature

Date	Medication Quantity Remaining	Authorized Signature

Disposition of Unused Drug

Date	Disposition Method / Notes	Authorized Signature

PATIENT NARCOTIC'S LOG

Page Start Date	From Page #	To Page #

Patient Information

Last Name	First Name	Middle Name/Init.	Room #	Bed#

Medication Name	Rx #	Prescribing Physician

☐ Oral	☐ Hypo	☐ Rectal	Initial Quantity Rec'd	Date Received	Pharmacy

Dosage / Directions

#	Date	Time	On Hand	Quantity Given	Rem-aining	From RX	Nurse Signature	Verified By Signature	Date	Time	Notes
1											
2											
3											
4											
5											
6											
7											
8											
9											
10											
11											
12											
13											
14											
15											
16											

Drug Depleted?	Date	Time	Signature

Date	Medication Quantity Remaining	Authorized Signature

Disposition of Unused Drug

Date	Disposition Method / Notes	Authorized Signature

PATIENT NARCOTIC'S LOG

Patient Information

Last Name	First Name	Middle Name/Init.	Room #	Bed#

Medication Name	Rx #	Prescribing Physician

☐ Oral ☐ Hypo ☐ Rectal

Initial Quantity Rec'd	Date Received	Pharmacy

Dosage / Directions

#	Date	Time	On Hand	Given	Quantity Remaining	From RX	Nurse Signature	Verified By Signature	Date	Time	Notes
1											
2											
3											
4											
5											
6											
7											
8											
9											
10											
11											
12											
13											
14											
15											
16											

Drug Depleted?	Date	Time	Signature

Date	Medication Quantity Remaining	Authorized Signature

Disposition of Unused Drug

Date	Disposition Method / Notes	Authorized Signature

PATIENT NARCOTIC'S LOG

Page Start Date	From Page #	To Page #

Patient Information

Last Name	First Name	Middle Name/Init.	Room #	Bed#

Medication Name	Rx #	Prescribing Physician

☐	☐	☐	Initial Quantity Rec'd	Date Received	Pharmacy
Oral	Hypo	Rectal			

Dosage / Directions

#	Date	Time	Quantity On Hand	Quantity Given	Quantity Rem-aining	Quantity From RX	Nurse Signature	Verified By Signature	Date	Time	Notes
1											
2											
3											
4											
5											
6											
7											
8											
9											
10											
11											
12											
13											
14											
15											
16											

Drug Depleted?	Date	Time	Signature

Date	Medication Quantity Remaining	Authorized Signature

Disposition of Unused Drug

Date	Disposition Method / Notes	Authorized Signature

PATIENT NARCOTIC'S LOG

Page Start Date	From Page #	To Page #

Patient Information

Last Name	First Name	Middle Name/Init.	Room #	Bed#

Medication Name	Rx #	Prescribing Physician

☐ Oral	☐ Hypo	☐ Rectal	Initial Quantity Rec'd	Date Received	Pharmacy

Dosage / Directions

#	Date	Time	On Hand	Given	Remaining	From RX	Nurse Signature	Verified By Signature	Date	Time	Notes
1											
2											
3											
4											
5											
6											
7											
8											
9											
10											
11											
12											
13											
14											
15											
16											

Drug Depleted?	Date	Time	Signature

Date	Medication Quantity Remaining	Authorized Signature

Disposition of Unused Drug		

Date	Disposition Method / Notes	Authorized Signature

PATIENT NARCOTIC'S LOG

Page Start Date	From Page #	To Page #

Patient Information

Last Name	First Name	Middle Name/Init.	Room # Bed#

Medication Name	Rx #	Prescribing Physician

☐ Oral ☐ Hypo ☐ Rectal	Initial Quantity Rec'd	Date Received	Pharmacy

Dosage / Directions

#	Date	Time	On Hand	Quantity Given	Quantity Rem-aining	From RX	Nurse Signature	Verified By Signature	Date	Time	Notes
1											
2											
3											
4											
5											
6											
7											
8											
9											
10											
11											
12											
13											
14											
15											
16											

Drug Depleted?	Date	Time	Signature

Date	Medication Quantity Remaining	Authorized Signature

Disposition of Unused Drug

Date	Disposition Method / Notes	Authorized Signature

PATIENT NARCOTIC'S LOG

Page Start Date	From Page #	To Page #

Patient Information

Last Name	First Name	Middle Name/Init.	Room #	Bed#

Medication Name	Rx #	Prescribing Physician

			Initial Quantity Rec'd		Date Received	Pharmacy
☐	☐	☐				
Oral	Hypo	Rectal				

Dosage / Directions

#	Date	Time	Quantity				Nurse Signature	Verified By Signature	Date	Time	Notes
			On Hand	Given	Rem-aining	From RX					
1											
2											
3											
4											
5											
6											
7											
8											
9											
10											
11											
12											
13											
14											
15											
16											

Drug Depleted?	Date	Time	Signature

Date	Medication Quantity Remaining	Authorized Signature

Disposition of Unused Drug

Date	Disposition Method / Notes	Authorized Signature

PATIENT NARCOTIC'S LOG

Page Start Date	From Page #	To Page #

Patient Information

Last Name	First Name	Middle Name/Init.	Room #	Bed#

Medication Name	Rx #	Prescribing Physician

☐ Oral	☐ Hypo	☐ Rectal	Initial Quantity Rec'd	Date Received	Pharmacy

Dosage / Directions

#	Date	Time	On Hand	Given	Rem-aining	From RX	Nurse Signature	Verified By Signature	Date	Time	Notes
1											
2											
3											
4											
5											
6											
7											
8											
9											
10											
11											
12											
13											
14											
15											
16											

Drug Depleted?	Date	Time	Signature

Date	Medication Quantity Remaining	Authorized Signature

Disposition of Unused Drug

Date	Disposition Method / Notes	Authorized Signature

PATIENT NARCOTIC'S LOG

Page Start Date	From Page #	To Page #

Patient Information

Last Name	First Name	Middle Name/Init.	Room #	Bed#

Medication Name	Rx #	Prescribing Physician

☐	☐	☐	Initial Quantity Rec'd	Date Received	Pharmacy
Oral	Hypo	Rectal			

Dosage / Directions

#	Date	Time	On Hand	Given	Quantity Rem-aining	From RX	Nurse Signature	Verified By Signature	Date	Time	Notes
1											
2											
3											
4											
5											
6											
7											
8											
9											
10											
11											
12											
13											
14											
15											
16											

Drug Depleted?	Date	Time	Signature

Date	Medication Quantity Remaining	Authorized Signature

Disposition of Unused Drug

Date	Disposition Method / Notes	Authorized Signature

PATIENT NARCOTIC'S LOG

Page Start Date	From Page #	To Page #

Patient Information

Last Name	First Name	Middle Name/Init.	Room #	Bed#

Medication Name	Rx #	Prescribing Physician

			Initial Quantity Rec'd	Date Received	Pharmacy
☐ Oral	☐ Hypo	☐ Rectal			

Dosage / Directions

#	Date	Time	Quantity On Hand	Quantity Given	Quantity Rem-aining	Quantity From RX	Nurse Signature	Verified By Signature	Date	Time	Notes
1											
2											
3											
4											
5											
6											
7											
8											
9											
10											
11											
12											
13											
14											
15											
16											

Drug Depleted?	Date	Time	Signature

Date	Medication Quantity Remaining	Authorized Signature

Disposition of Unused Drug

Date	Disposition Method / Notes	Authorized Signature

PATIENT NARCOTIC'S LOG

Page Start Date	From Page #	To Page #

Patient Information

Last Name	First Name	Middle Name/Init.	Room #	Bed#

Medication Name	Rx #	Prescribing Physician

			Initial Quantity Rec'd	Date Received	Pharmacy
☐	☐	☐			
Oral	Hypo	Rectal			

Dosage / Directions

#	Date	Time	On Hand	Given	Rem-aining	From RX	Nurse Signature	Verified By Signature	Date	Time	Notes
					Quantity						
1											
2											
3											
4											
5											
6											
7											
8											
9											
10											
11											
12											
13											
14											
15											
16											

Drug Depleted?	Date	Time	Signature

Date	Medication Quantity Remaining	Authorized Signature

Disposition of Unused Drug

Date	Disposition Method / Notes	Authorized Signature

PATIENT NARCOTIC'S LOG

Page Start Date	From Page #	To Page #

Patient Information

Last Name	First Name	Middle Name/Init.	Room #	Bed#

Medication Name	Rx #	Prescribing Physician

			Initial Quantity Rec'd	Date Received	Pharmacy
☐ Oral	☐ Hypo	☐ Rectal			

Dosage / Directions

#	Date	Time	On Hand	Quantity Given	Rem-aining	From RX	Nurse Signature	Verified By Signature	Date	Time	Notes
1											
2											
3											
4											
5											
6											
7											
8											
9											
10											
11											
12											
13											
14											
15											
16											

Drug Depleted?	Date	Time	Signature

Date	Medication Quantity Remaining	Authorized Signature

Disposition of Unused Drug

Date	Disposition Method / Notes	Authorized Signature

PATIENT NARCOTIC'S LOG

Page Start Date	From Page #	To Page #

Patient Information

Last Name	First Name	Middle Name/Init. Room #	Bed#

Medication Name	Rx #	Prescribing Physician

☐ Oral	☐ Hypo	☐ Rectal	Initial Quantity Rec'd	Date Received	Pharmacy

Dosage / Directions

#	Date	Time	On Hand	Quantity Given	Quantity Rem-aining	From RX	Nurse Signature	Verified By Signature	Date	Time	Notes
1											
2											
3											
4											
5											
6											
7											
8											
9											
10											
11											
12											
13											
14											
15											
16											

Drug Depleted?	Date	Time	Signature

Date	Medication Quantity Remaining	Authorized Signature

Disposition of Unused Drug

Date	Disposition Method / Notes	Authorized Signature

PATIENT NARCOTIC'S LOG

Page Start Date	From Page #	To Page #

Patient Information

Last Name	First Name	Middle Name/Init.	Room #	Bed#

Medication Name	Rx #	Prescribing Physician

☐ Oral	☐ Hypo	☐ Rectal	Initial Quantity Rec'd	Date Received	Pharmacy

Dosage / Directions

#	Date	Time	On Hand	Quantity Given	Quantity Rem-aining	From RX	Nurse Signature	Verified By Signature	Date	Time	Notes
1											
2											
3											
4											
5											
6											
7											
8											
9											
10											
11											
12											
13											
14											
15											
16											

Drug Depleted?	Date	Time	Signature

Date	Medication Quantity Remaining	Authorized Signature

Disposition of Unused Drug

Date	Disposition Method / Notes	Authorized Signature

PATIENT NARCOTIC'S LOG

Page Start Date	From Page #	To Page #

Patient Information

Last Name	First Name	Middle Name/Init.	Room #	Bed#

Medication Name	Rx #	Prescribing Physician

☐ Oral	☐ Hypo	☐ Rectal	Initial Quantity Rec'd	Date Received	Pharmacy

Dosage / Directions

#	Date	Time	On Hand	Quantity Given	Quantity Rem-aining	From RX	Nurse Signature	Verified By Signature	Date	Time	Notes
1											
2											
3											
4											
5											
6											
7											
8											
9											
10											
11											
12											
13											
14											
15											
16											

Drug Depleted?	Date	Time	Signature

Date	Medication Quantity Remaining	Authorized Signature

Disposition of Unused Drug

Date	Disposition Method / Notes	Authorized Signature

PATIENT NARCOTIC'S LOG

Page Start Date	From Page #	To Page #

Patient Information

Last Name	First Name	Middle Name/Init.	Room #	Bed#

Medication Name	Rx #	Prescribing Physician

☐ Oral	☐ Hypo	☐ Rectal	Initial Quantity Rec'd	Date Received	Pharmacy

Dosage / Directions

#	Date	Time	On Hand	Quantity Given	Quantity Rem-aining	From RX	Nurse Signature	Verified By Signature	Date	Time	Notes
1											
2											
3											
4											
5											
6											
7											
8											
9											
10											
11											
12											
13											
14											
15											
16											

Drug Depleted?	Date	Time	Signature

Date	Medication Quantity Remaining	Authorized Signature

Disposition of Unused Drug

Date	Disposition Method / Notes	Authorized Signature

PATIENT NARCOTIC'S LOG

	Page Start Date	From Page #	To Page #

Patient Information

Last Name	First Name	Middle Name/Init.	Room #	Bed#

Medication Name	Rx #	Prescribing Physician

☐	☐	☐	Initial Quantity Rec'd	Date Received	Pharmacy
Oral	Hypo	Rectal			

Dosage / Directions

#	Date	Time	On Hand	Quantity Given	Rem-aining	From RX	Nurse Signature	Verified By Signature	Date	Time	Notes
1											
2											
3											
4											
5											
6											
7											
8											
9											
10											
11											
12											
13											
14											
15											
16											

Drug Depleted?	Date	Time	Signature

Date	Medication Quantity Remaining	Authorized Signature

Disposition of Unused Drug

Date	Disposition Method / Notes	Authorized Signature

PATIENT NARCOTIC'S LOG

Page Start Date	From Page #	To Page #

Patient Information

Last Name	First Name	Middle Name/Init.	Room #	Bed#

Medication Name	Rx #	Prescribing Physician

☐	☐	☐	Initial Quantity Rec'd	Date Received	Pharmacy
Oral	Hypo	Rectal			

Dosage / Directions

#	Date	Time	Quantity On Hand	Quantity Given	Quantity Rem-aining	Quantity From RX	Nurse Signature	Verified By Signature	Date	Time	Notes
1											
2											
3											
4											
5											
6											
7											
8											
9											
10											
11											
12											
13											
14											
15											
16											

Drug Depleted?	Date	Time	Signature

Date	Medication Quantity Remaining	Authorized Signature

Disposition of Unused Drug

Date	Disposition Method / Notes	Authorized Signature

PATIENT NARCOTIC'S LOG

Page Start Date	From Page #	To Page #

Patient Information

Last Name	First Name	Middle Name/Init. Room #	Bed#

Medication Name	Rx #	Prescribing Physician

☐ Oral ☐ Hypo ☐ Rectal	Initial Quantity Rec'd	Date Received	Pharmacy

Dosage / Directions

#	Date	Time	On Hand	Quantity Given	Quantity Rem-aining	From RX	Nurse Signature	Verified By Signature	Date	Time	Notes
1											
2											
3											
4											
5											
6											
7											
8											
9											
10											
11											
12											
13											
14											
15											
16											

Drug Depleted?	Date	Time	Signature

Date	Medication Quantity Remaining	Authorized Signature

Disposition of Unused Drug

Date	Disposition Method / Notes	Authorized Signature

PATIENT NARCOTIC'S LOG

Patient Information

Last Name	First Name	Middle Name/Init.	Room #	Bed#

Medication Name	Rx #	Prescribing Physician

☐ Oral	☐ Hypo	☐ Rectal	Initial Quantity Rec'd	Date Received	Pharmacy

Dosage / Directions

#	Date	Time	Quantity On Hand	Quantity Given	Quantity Rem-aining	Quantity From RX	Nurse Signature	Verified By Signature	Date	Time	Notes
1											
2											
3											
4											
5											
6											
7											
8											
9											
10											
11											
12											
13											
14											
15											
16											

Drug Depleted?	Date	Time	Signature

Date	Medication Quantity Remaining	Authorized Signature

Disposition of Unused Drug

Date	Disposition Method / Notes	Authorized Signature

PATIENT NARCOTIC'S LOG

Page Start Date	From Page #	To Page #

Patient Information

Last Name	First Name	Middle Name/Init.	Room #	Bed#

Medication Name	Rx #	Prescribing Physician

☐ Oral	☐ Hypo	☐ Rectal	Initial Quantity Rec'd	Date Received	Pharmacy

Dosage / Directions

#	Date	Time	On Hand	Quantity Given	Quantity Rem-aining	From RX	Nurse Signature	Verified By Signature	Date	Time	Notes
1											
2											
3											
4											
5											
6											
7											
8											
9											
10											
11											
12											
13											
14											
15											
16											

Drug Depleted?	Date	Time	Signature

Date	Medication Quantity Remaining	Authorized Signature

Disposition of Unused Drug

Date	Disposition Method / Notes	Authorized Signature

PATIENT NARCOTIC'S LOG

Page Start Date	From Page #	To Page #

Patient Information

Last Name	First Name	Middle Name/Init.	Room #	Bed#

Medication Name	Rx #	Prescribing Physician

☐ Oral	☐ Hypo	☐ Rectal	Initial Quantity Rec'd	Date Received	Pharmacy

Dosage / Directions

#	Date	Time	Quantity On Hand	Quantity Given	Quantity Rem-aining	Quantity From RX	Nurse Signature	Verified By Signature	Date	Time	Notes
1											
2											
3											
4											
5											
6											
7											
8											
9											
10											
11											
12											
13											
14											
15											
16											

Drug Depleted?	Date	Time	Signature

Date	Medication Quantity Remaining	Authorized Signature

Disposition of Unused Drug

Date	Disposition Method / Notes	Authorized Signature

PATIENT NARCOTIC'S LOG

Page Start Date	From Page #	To Page #

Patient Information

Last Name	First Name	Middle Name/Init.	Room #	Bed#

Medication Name	Rx #	Prescribing Physician

☐ Oral	☐ Hypo	☐ Rectal	Initial Quantity Rec'd	Date Received	Pharmacy

Dosage / Directions

#	Date	Time	On Hand	Quantity Given	Quantity Rem-aining	From RX	Nurse Signature	Verified By Signature	Date	Time	Notes
1											
2											
3											
4											
5											
6											
7											
8											
9											
10											
11											
12											
13											
14											
15											
16											

Drug Depleted?	Date	Time	Signature

Date	Medication Quantity Remaining	Authorized Signature

Disposition of Unused Drug

Date	Disposition Method / Notes	Authorized Signature

PATIENT NARCOTIC'S LOG

Page Start Date	From Page #	To Page #

Patient Information

Last Name	First Name	Middle Name/Init.	Room #	Bed#

Medication Name	Rx #	Prescribing Physician

			Initial Quantity Rec'd	Date Received	Pharmacy
☐ Oral	☐ Hypo	☐ Rectal			

Dosage / Directions

#	Date	Time	Quantity On Hand	Quantity Given	Quantity Rem-aining	From RX	Nurse Signature	Verified By Signature	Date	Time	Notes
1											
2											
3											
4											
5											
6											
7											
8											
9											
10											
11											
12											
13											
14											
15											
16											

Drug Depleted?	Date	Time	Signature

Date	Medication Quantity Remaining	Authorized Signature

Disposition of Unused Drug

Date	Disposition Method / Notes	Authorized Signature

PATIENT NARCOTIC'S LOG

Page Start Date	From Page #	To Page #

Patient Information

Last Name	First Name	Middle Name/Init. Room #	Bed#

Medication Name	Rx #	Prescribing Physician

☐ Oral	☐ Hypo	☐ Rectal	Initial Quantity Rec'd	Date Received	Pharmacy

Dosage / Directions

#	Date	Time	On Hand	Quantity Given	Quantity Rem-aining	From RX	Nurse Signature	Verified By Signature	Date	Time	Notes
1											
2											
3											
4											
5											
6											
7											
8											
9											
10											
11											
12											
13											
14											
15											
16											

Drug Depleted?	Date	Time	Signature

Date	Medication Quantity Remaining	Authorized Signature

Disposition of Unused Drug

Date	Disposition Method / Notes	Authorized Signature

PATIENT NARCOTIC'S LOG

Page Start Date	From Page #	To Page #

Patient Information

Last Name	First Name	Middle Name/Init.	Room # Bed#

Medication Name	Rx #	Prescribing Physician

☐ Oral ☐ Hypo ☐ Rectal	Initial Quantity Rec'd	Date Received	Pharmacy

Dosage / Directions

#	Date	Time	Quantity On Hand	Quantity Given	Quantity Rem-aining	Quantity From RX	Nurse Signature	Verified By Signature	Date	Time	Notes
1											
2											
3											
4											
5											
6											
7											
8											
9											
10											
11											
12											
13											
14											
15											
16											

Drug Depleted?	Date	Time	Signature

Date	Medication Quantity Remaining	Authorized Signature

Disposition of Unused Drug

Date	Disposition Method / Notes	Authorized Signature

PATIENT NARCOTIC'S LOG

Page Start Date	From Page #	To Page #

Patient Information

Last Name	First Name	Middle Name/Init.	Room #	Bed#

Medication Name	Rx #	Prescribing Physician

☐ Oral	☐ Hypo	☐ Rectal	Initial Quantity Rec'd	Date Received	Pharmacy

Dosage / Directions

#	Date	Time	On Hand	Given	Remaining	From RX	Nurse Signature	Verified By Signature	Date	Time	Notes
1											
2											
3											
4											
5											
6											
7											
8											
9											
10											
11											
12											
13											
14											
15											
16											

Quantity (spanning On Hand, Given, Remaining, From RX)

Drug Depleted?	Date	Time	Signature

Date	Medication Quantity Remaining	Authorized Signature

Disposition of Unused Drug

Date	Disposition Method / Notes	Authorized Signature

PATIENT NARCOTIC'S LOG

<table>
<tr><td colspan="3">Page Start Date</td><td>From Page #</td><td>To Page #</td></tr>
</table>

Patient Information

Last Name	First Name	Middle Name/Init.	Room #	Bed#

Medication Name	Rx #	Prescribing Physician

☐ Oral ☐ Hypo ☐ Rectal

Initial Quantity Rec'd	Date Received	Pharmacy

Dosage / Directions

#	Date	Time	Quantity On Hand	Quantity Given	Quantity Rem-aining	From RX	Nurse Signature	Verified By Signature	Date	Time	Notes
1											
2											
3											
4											
5											
6											
7											
8											
9											
10											
11											
12											
13											
14											
15											
16											

Drug Depleted?	Date	Time	Signature

Date	Medication Quantity Remaining	Authorized Signature

Disposition of Unused Drug

Date	Disposition Method / Notes	Authorized Signature

PATIENT NARCOTIC'S LOG

Page Start Date	From Page #	To Page #

Patient Information

Last Name	First Name	Middle Name/Init.	Room #	Bed#

Medication Name	Rx #	Prescribing Physician

☐ Oral	☐ Hypo	☐ Rectal	Initial Quantity Rec'd	Date Received	Pharmacy

Dosage / Directions

#	Date	Time	On Hand	Given	Rem-aining	From RX	Nurse Signature	Verified By Signature	Date	Time	Notes
1											
2											
3											
4											
5											
6											
7											
8											
9											
10											
11											
12											
13											
14											
15											
16											

Drug Depleted?	Date	Time	Signature

Date	Medication Quantity Remaining	Authorized Signature

Disposition of Unused Drug		
Date	Disposition Method / Notes	Authorized Signature

PATIENT NARCOTIC'S LOG

Patient Information

Last Name	First Name	Middle Name/Init.	Room #	Bed#

Medication Name	Rx #	Prescribing Physician

			Initial Quantity Rec'd	Date Received	Pharmacy
☐ Oral	☐ Hypo	☐ Rectal			

Dosage / Directions

#	Date	Time	On Hand	Quantity Given	Quantity Rem-aining	Quantity From RX	Nurse Signature	Verified By Signature	Date	Time	Notes
1											
2											
3											
4											
5											
6											
7											
8											
9											
10											
11											
12											
13											
14											
15											
16											

Drug Depleted?	Date	Time	Signature

Date	Medication Quantity Remaining	Authorized Signature

Disposition of Unused Drug

Date	Disposition Method / Notes	Authorized Signature

PATIENT NARCOTIC'S LOG

Page Start Date	From Page #	To Page #

Patient Information

Last Name	First Name	Middle Name/Init.	Room #	Bed#

Medication Name	Rx #	Prescribing Physician

☐ Oral	☐ Hypo	☐ Rectal	Initial Quantity Rec'd	Date Received	Pharmacy

Dosage / Directions

#	Date	Time	Quantity On Hand	Quantity Given	Quantity Rem-aining	From RX	Nurse Signature	Verified By Signature	Date	Time	Notes
1											
2											
3											
4											
5											
6											
7											
8											
9											
10											
11											
12											
13											
14											
15											
16											

Drug Depleted?	Date	Time	Signature

Date	Medication Quantity Remaining	Authorized Signature

Disposition of Unused Drug

Date	Disposition Method / Notes	Authorized Signature

PATIENT NARCOTIC'S LOG

Page Start Date	From Page #	To Page #

Patient Information

Last Name	First Name	Middle Name/Init.	Room #	Bed#

Medication Name	Rx #	Prescribing Physician

☐	☐	☐	Initial Quantity Rec'd	Date Received	Pharmacy
Oral	Hypo	Rectal			

Dosage / Directions

#	Date	Time	On Hand	Quantity Given	Quantity Rem-aining	From RX	Nurse Signature	Verified By Signature	Date	Time	Notes
1											
2											
3											
4											
5											
6											
7											
8											
9											
10											
11											
12											
13											
14											
15											
16											

Drug Depleted?	Date	Time	Signature

Date	Medication Quantity Remaining	Authorized Signature

Disposition of Unused Drug

Date	Disposition Method / Notes	Authorized Signature

PATIENT NARCOTIC'S LOG

Page Start Date	From Page #	To Page #

Patient Information

Last Name	First Name	Middle Name/Init.	Room #	Bed#

Medication Name	Rx #	Prescribing Physician

☐ Oral	☐ Hypo	☐ Rectal	Initial Quantity Rec'd	Date Received	Pharmacy

Dosage / Directions

#	Date	Time	On Hand	Quantity Given	Quantity Rem-aining	From RX	Nurse Signature	Verified By Signature	Date	Time	Notes
1											
2											
3											
4											
5											
6											
7											
8											
9											
10											
11											
12											
13											
14											
15											
16											

Drug Depleted?	Date	Time	Signature

Date	Medication Quantity Remaining	Authorized Signature

Disposition of Unused Drug

Date	Disposition Method / Notes	Authorized Signature

PATIENT NARCOTIC'S LOG

Page Start Date	From Page #	To Page #

Patient Information

Last Name	First Name	Middle Name/Init.	Room #	Bed#

Medication Name	Rx #	Prescribing Physician

☐ Oral ☐ Hypo ☐ Rectal

Initial Quantity Rec'd	Date Received	Pharmacy

Dosage / Directions

#	Date	Time	On Hand	Given	Quantity Rem-aining	From RX	Nurse Signature	Verified By Signature	Date	Time	Notes
1											
2											
3											
4											
5											
6											
7											
8											
9											
10											
11											
12											
13											
14											
15											
16											

Drug Depleted?	Date	Time	Signature

Date	Medication Quantity Remaining	Authorized Signature

Disposition of Unused Drug

Date	Disposition Method / Notes	Authorized Signature

PATIENT NARCOTIC'S LOG

Patient Information

| Last Name | First Name | Middle Name/Init. | Room # | Bed# |

| Medication Name | Rx # | Prescribing Physician |

| ☐ Oral | ☐ Hypo | ☐ Rectal | Initial Quantity Rec'd | Date Received | Pharmacy |

Dosage / Directions

#	Date	Time	On Hand	Given	Rem-aining	From RX	Nurse Signature	Verified By Signature	Date	Time	Notes
			Quantity								
1											
2											
3											
4											
5											
6											
7											
8											
9											
10											
11											
12											
13											
14											
15											
16											

| Drug Depleted? | Date | Time | Signature |

| Date | Medication Quantity Remaining | Authorized Signature |

Disposition of Unused Drug

| Date | Disposition Method / Notes | Authorized Signature |

PATIENT NARCOTIC'S LOG

Page Start Date	From Page #	To Page #

Patient Information

Last Name	First Name	Middle Name/Init.	Room #	Bed#

Medication Name	Rx #	Prescribing Physician

Oral	Hypo	Rectal	Initial Quantity Rec'd	Date Received	Pharmacy
☐	☐	☐			

Dosage / Directions

#	Date	Time	Quantity On Hand	Quantity Given	Quantity Rem-aining	Quantity From RX	Nurse Signature	Verified By Signature	Date	Time	Notes
1											
2											
3											
4											
5											
6											
7											
8											
9											
10											
11											
12											
13											
14											
15											
16											

Drug Depleted?	Date	Time	Signature

Date	Medication Quantity Remaining	Authorized Signature

Disposition of Unused Drug

Date	Disposition Method / Notes	Authorized Signature

PATIENT NARCOTIC'S LOG

Page Start Date	From Page #	To Page #

Patient Information

Last Name	First Name	Middle Name/Init.	Room #	Bed#

Medication Name	Rx #	Prescribing Physician

☐ Oral ☐ Hypo ☐ Rectal	Initial Quantity Rec'd	Date Received	Pharmacy

Dosage / Directions

#	Date	Time	Quantity On Hand	Quantity Given	Quantity Rem-aining	Quantity From RX	Nurse Signature	Verified By Signature	Date	Time	Notes
1											
2											
3											
4											
5											
6											
7											
8											
9											
10											
11											
12											
13											
14											
15											
16											

Drug Depleted?	Date	Time	Signature

Date	Medication Quantity Remaining	Authorized Signature

Disposition of Unused Drug

Date	Disposition Method / Notes	Authorized Signature

PATIENT NARCOTIC'S LOG

Page Start Date	From Page #	To Page #

Patient Information

Last Name	First Name	Middle Name/Init.	Room #	Bed#

Medication Name	Rx #	Prescribing Physician

☐ Oral	☐ Hypo	☐ Rectal	Initial Quantity Rec'd	Date Received	Pharmacy

Dosage / Directions

#	Date	Time	Quantity On Hand	Quantity Given	Quantity Rem-aining	Quantity From RX	Nurse Signature	Verified By Signature	Date	Time	Notes
1											
2											
3											
4											
5											
6											
7											
8											
9											
10											
11											
12											
13											
14											
15											
16											

Drug Depleted?	Date	Time	Signature

Date	Medication Quantity Remaining	Authorized Signature

Disposition of Unused Drug

Date	Disposition Method / Notes	Authorized Signature

PATIENT NARCOTIC'S LOG

Page Start Date	From Page #	To Page #

Patient Information

Last Name	First Name	Middle Name/Init.	Room #	Bed#

Medication Name	Rx #	Prescribing Physician

☐ Oral	☐ Hypo	☐ Rectal	Initial Quantity Rec'd	Date Received	Pharmacy

Dosage / Directions

#	Date	Time	On Hand	Quantity Given	Quantity Rem-aining	From RX	Nurse Signature	Verified By Signature	Date	Time	Notes
1											
2											
3											
4											
5											
6											
7											
8											
9											
10											
11											
12											
13											
14											
15											
16											

Drug Depleted?	Date	Time	Signature

Date	Medication Quantity Remaining	Authorized Signature

Disposition of Unused Drug

Date	Disposition Method / Notes	Authorized Signature

PATIENT NARCOTIC'S LOG

Page Start Date	From Page #	To Page #

Patient Information

Last Name	First Name	Middle Name/Init.	Room #	Bed#

Medication Name	Rx #	Prescribing Physician

			Initial Quantity Rec'd	Date Received	Pharmacy
☐ Oral	☐ Hypo	☐ Rectal			

Dosage / Directions

#	Date	Time	On Hand	Quantity Given	Quantity Rem-aining	From RX	Nurse Signature	Verified By Signature	Date	Time	Notes
1											
2											
3											
4											
5											
6											
7											
8											
9											
10											
11											
12											
13											
14											
15											
16											

Drug Depleted?	Date	Time	Signature

Date	Medication Quantity Remaining	Authorized Signature

Disposition of Unused Drug

Date	Disposition Method / Notes	Authorized Signature

PATIENT NARCOTIC'S LOG

Page Start Date	From Page #	To Page #

Patient Information

Last Name	First Name	Middle Name/Init.	Room #	Bed#

Medication Name	Rx #	Prescribing Physician

☐ Oral	☐ Hypo	☐ Rectal	Initial Quantity Rec'd	Date Received	Pharmacy

Dosage / Directions

#	Date	Time	On Hand	Given	Rem-aining	From RX	Nurse Signature	Verified By Signature	Date	Time	Notes
				Quantity							
1											
2											
3											
4											
5											
6											
7											
8											
9											
10											
11											
12											
13											
14											
15											
16											

Drug Depleted?	Date	Time	Signature

Date	Medication Quantity Remaining	Authorized Signature

Disposition of Unused Drug

Date	Disposition Method / Notes	Authorized Signature

PATIENT NARCOTIC'S LOG

Page Start Date	From Page #	To Page #

Patient Information

Last Name	First Name	Middle Name/Init.	Room #	Bed#

Medication Name	Rx #	Prescribing Physician

☐ Oral	☐ Hypo	☐ Rectal	Initial Quantity Rec'd	Date Received	Pharmacy

Dosage / Directions

#	Date	Time	On Hand	Quantity Given	Quantity Rem-aining	From RX	Nurse Signature	Verified By Signature	Date	Time	Notes
1											
2											
3											
4											
5											
6											
7											
8											
9											
10											
11											
12											
13											
14											
15											
16											

Drug Depleted?	Date	Time	Signature

Date	Medication Quantity Remaining	Authorized Signature

Disposition of Unused Drug

Date	Disposition Method / Notes	Authorized Signature

PATIENT NARCOTIC'S LOG

Page Start Date	From Page #	To Page #

Patient Information

Last Name	First Name	Middle Name/Init.	Room #	Bed#

Medication Name	Rx #	Prescribing Physician

☐ Oral	☐ Hypo	☐ Rectal	Initial Quantity Rec'd	Date Received	Pharmacy

Dosage / Directions

#	Date	Time	On Hand	Quantity Given	Quantity Rem-aining	From RX	Nurse Signature	Verified By Signature	Date	Time	Notes
1											
2											
3											
4											
5											
6											
7											
8											
9											
10											
11											
12											
13											
14											
15											
16											

Drug Depleted?	Date	Time	Signature

Date	Medication Quantity Remaining	Authorized Signature

Disposition of Unused Drug

Date	Disposition Method / Notes	Authorized Signature

PATIENT NARCOTIC'S LOG

Page Start Date	From Page #	To Page #

Patient Information

Last Name	First Name	Middle Name/Init.	Room #	Bed#

Medication Name	Rx #	Prescribing Physician

☐ Oral	☐ Hypo	☐ Rectal	Initial Quantity Rec'd	Date Received	Pharmacy

Dosage / Directions

#	Date	Time	Quantity On Hand	Given	Rem-aining	From RX	Nurse Signature	Verified By Signature	Date	Time	Notes
1											
2											
3											
4											
5											
6											
7											
8											
9											
10											
11											
12											
13											
14											
15											
16											

Drug Depleted?	Date	Time	Signature

Date	Medication Quantity Remaining	Authorized Signature

Disposition of Unused Drug

Date	Disposition Method / Notes	Authorized Signature

PATIENT NARCOTIC'S LOG

Page Start Date	From Page #	To Page #

Patient Information

Last Name	First Name	Middle Name/Init.	Room #	Bed#

Medication Name	Rx #	Prescribing Physician

☐ Oral	☐ Hypo	☐ Rectal	Initial Quantity Rec'd	Date Received	Pharmacy

Dosage / Directions

#	Date	Time	On Hand	Quantity Given	Quantity Rem-aining	From RX	Nurse Signature	Verified By Signature	Date	Time	Notes
1											
2											
3											
4											
5											
6											
7											
8											
9											
10											
11											
12											
13											
14											
15											
16											

Drug Depleted?	Date	Time	Signature

Date	Medication Quantity Remaining	Authorized Signature

Disposition of Unused Drug

Date	Disposition Method / Notes	Authorized Signature

PATIENT NARCOTIC'S LOG

Page Start Date	From Page #	To Page #

Patient Information

Last Name	First Name	Middle Name/Init.	Room #	Bed#

Medication Name	Rx #	Prescribing Physician

☐ Oral	☐ Hypo	☐ Rectal	Initial Quantity Rec'd	Date Received	Pharmacy

Dosage / Directions

#	Date	Time	Quantity On Hand	Quantity Given	Quantity Rem-aining	Quantity From RX	Nurse Signature	Verified By Signature	Date	Time	Notes
1											
2											
3											
4											
5											
6											
7											
8											
9											
10											
11											
12											
13											
14											
15											
16											

Drug Depleted?	Date	Time	Signature

Date	Medication Quantity Remaining	Authorized Signature

Disposition of Unused Drug

Date	Disposition Method / Notes	Authorized Signature

PATIENT NARCOTIC'S LOG

Page Start Date	From Page #	To Page #

Patient Information

Last Name	First Name	Middle Name/Init.	Room #	Bed#

Medication Name	Rx #	Prescribing Physician

☐ Oral	☐ Hypo	☐ Rectal	Initial Quantity Rec'd	Date Received	Pharmacy

Dosage / Directions

#	Date	Time	On Hand	Quantity Given	Quantity Rem-aining	From RX	Nurse Signature	Verified By Signature	Date	Time	Notes
1											
2											
3											
4											
5											
6											
7											
8											
9											
10											
11											
12											
13											
14											
15											
16											

Drug Depleted?	Date	Time	Signature

Date	Medication Quantity Remaining	Authorized Signature

Disposition of Unused Drug

Date	Disposition Method / Notes	Authorized Signature

PATIENT NARCOTIC'S LOG

Page Start Date	From Page #	To Page #

Patient Information

Last Name	First Name	Middle Name/Init.	Room #	Bed#

Medication Name	Rx #	Prescribing Physician

☐ Oral	☐ Hypo	☐ Rectal	Initial Quantity Rec'd	Date Received	Pharmacy

Dosage / Directions

#	Date	Time	Quantity On Hand	Quantity Given	Quantity Rem-aining	From RX	Nurse Signature	Verified By Signature	Date	Time	Notes
1											
2											
3											
4											
5											
6											
7											
8											
9											
10											
11											
12											
13											
14											
15											
16											

Drug Depleted?	Date	Time	Signature

Date	Medication Quantity Remaining	Authorized Signature

Disposition of Unused Drug

Date	Disposition Method / Notes	Authorized Signature

PATIENT NARCOTIC'S LOG

Page Start Date	From Page #	To Page #

Patient Information

Last Name	First Name	Middle Name/Init.	Room #	Bed#

Medication Name	Rx #	Prescribing Physician

☐ Oral	☐ Hypo	☐ Rectal	Initial Quantity Rec'd	Date Received	Pharmacy

Dosage / Directions

#	Date	Time	On Hand	Quantity Given	Rem-aining	From RX	Nurse Signature	Verified By Signature	Date	Time	Notes
1											
2											
3											
4											
5											
6											
7											
8											
9											
10											
11											
12											
13											
14											
15											
16											

Drug Depleted?	Date	Time	Signature

Date	Medication Quantity Remaining	Authorized Signature

Disposition of Unused Drug

Date	Disposition Method / Notes	Authorized Signature

PATIENT NARCOTIC'S LOG

	Page Start Date	From Page #	To Page #

Patient Information

Last Name	First Name	Middle Name/Init.	Room #	Bed#

Medication Name	Rx #	Prescribing Physician

☐ Oral	☐ Hypo	☐ Rectal	Initial Quantity Rec'd	Date Received	Pharmacy

Dosage / Directions

#	Date	Time	Quantity On Hand	Quantity Given	Quantity Rem-aining	Quantity From RX	Nurse Signature	Verified By Signature	Date	Time	Notes
1											
2											
3											
4											
5											
6											
7											
8											
9											
10											
11											
12											
13											
14											
15											
16											

Drug Depleted?	Date	Time	Signature

Date	Medication Quantity Remaining	Authorized Signature

Disposition of Unused Drug		

Date	Disposition Method / Notes	Authorized Signature

PATIENT NARCOTIC'S LOG

Patient Information

| Last Name | First Name | Middle Name/Init. | Room # | Bed# |

| Medication Name | Rx # | Prescribing Physician |

| ☐ | ☐ | ☐ | Initial Quantity Rec'd | Date Received | Pharmacy |
| Oral | Hypo | Rectal | | | |

Dosage / Directions

#	Date	Time	On Hand	Quantity Given	Quantity Rem-aining	From RX	Nurse Signature	Verified By Signature	Date	Time	Notes
1											
2											
3											
4											
5											
6											
7											
8											
9											
10											
11											
12											
13											
14											
15											
16											

| Drug Depleted? | Date | Time | Signature |

| Date | Medication Quantity Remaining | Authorized Signature |

Disposition of Unused Drug

| Date | Disposition Method / Notes | Authorized Signature |

PATIENT NARCOTIC'S LOG

Page Start Date	From Page #	To Page #

Patient Information

Last Name	First Name	Middle Name/Init.	Room #	Bed#

Medication Name	Rx #	Prescribing Physician

☐ Oral	☐ Hypo	☐ Rectal	Initial Quantity Rec'd	Date Received	Pharmacy

Dosage / Directions

#	Date	Time	On Hand	Given	Rem-aining	From RX	Nurse Signature	Verified By Signature	Date	Time	Notes
1											
2											
3											
4											
5											
6											
7											
8											
9											
10											
11											
12											
13											
14											
15											
16											

Quantity (Given / Remaining / From RX)

Drug Depleted?	Date	Time	Signature

Date	Medication Quantity Remaining	Authorized Signature

Disposition of Unused Drug

Date	Disposition Method / Notes	Authorized Signature

PATIENT NARCOTIC'S LOG

Page Start Date	From Page #	To Page #

Patient Information

Last Name	First Name	Middle Name/Init.	Room #	Bed#

Medication Name	Rx #	Prescribing Physician

☐ Oral	☐ Hypo	☐ Rectal	Initial Quantity Rec'd	Date Received	Pharmacy

Dosage / Directions

#	Date	Time	On Hand	Quantity Given	Quantity Rem-aining	From RX	Nurse Signature	Verified By Signature	Date	Time	Notes
1											
2											
3											
4											
5											
6											
7											
8											
9											
10											
11											
12											
13											
14											
15											
16											

Drug Depleted?	Date	Time	Signature

Date	Medication Quantity Remaining	Authorized Signature

Disposition of Unused Drug

Date	Disposition Method / Notes	Authorized Signature

PATIENT NARCOTIC'S LOG

Page Start Date	From Page #	To Page #

Patient Information

Last Name	First Name	Middle Name/Init.	Room # Bed#

Medication Name	Rx #	Prescribing Physician

☐ Oral ☐ Hypo ☐ Rectal	Initial Quantity Rec'd	Date Received	Pharmacy

Dosage / Directions

#	Date	Time	Quantity On Hand	Quantity Given	Quantity Rem-aining	Quantity From RX	Nurse Signature	Verified By Signature	Date	Time	Notes
1											
2											
3											
4											
5											
6											
7											
8											
9											
10											
11											
12											
13											
14											
15											
16											

Drug Depleted?	Date	Time	Signature

Date	Medication Quantity Remaining	Authorized Signature

Disposition of Unused Drug

Date	Disposition Method / Notes	Authorized Signature

PATIENT NARCOTIC'S LOG

Page Start Date	From Page #	To Page #

Patient Information

Last Name	First Name	Middle Name/Init.	Room #	Bed#

Medication Name	Rx #	Prescribing Physician

☐ Oral	☐ Hypo	☐ Rectal	Initial Quantity Rec'd	Date Received	Pharmacy

Dosage / Directions

#	Date	Time	On Hand	Quantity Given	Quantity Rem-aining	From RX	Nurse Signature	Verified By Signature	Date	Time	Notes
1											
2											
3											
4											
5											
6											
7											
8											
9											
10											
11											
12											
13											
14											
15											
16											

Drug Depleted?	Date	Time	Signature

Date	Medication Quantity Remaining	Authorized Signature

Disposition of Unused Drug

Date	Disposition Method / Notes	Authorized Signature

PATIENT NARCOTIC'S LOG

Page Start Date	From Page #	To Page #

Patient Information

Last Name	First Name	Middle Name/Init.	Room #	Bed#

Medication Name	Rx #	Prescribing Physician

☐ Oral   ☐ Hypo   ☐ Rectal

Initial Quantity Rec'd	Date Received	Pharmacy

Dosage / Directions

#	Date	Time	Quantity On Hand	Given	Rem-aining	From RX	Nurse Signature	Verified By Signature	Date	Time	Notes
1											
2											
3											
4											
5											
6											
7											
8											
9											
10											
11											
12											
13											
14											
15											
16											

Drug Depleted?	Date	Time	Signature

Date	Medication Quantity Remaining	Authorized Signature

Disposition of Unused Drug

Date	Disposition Method / Notes	Authorized Signature

PATIENT NARCOTIC'S LOG

Page Start Date	From Page #	To Page #

Patient Information

Last Name	First Name	Middle Name/Init.	Room #	Bed#

Medication Name	Rx #	Prescribing Physician

☐ Oral	☐ Hypo	☐ Rectal	Initial Quantity Rec'd	Date Received	Pharmacy

Dosage / Directions

#	Date	Time	On Hand	Given	Remaining	From RX	Nurse Signature	Verified By Signature	Date	Time	Notes
1											
2											
3											
4											
5											
6											
7											
8											
9											
10											
11											
12											
13											
14											
15											
16											

Drug Depleted?	Date	Time	Signature

Date	Medication Quantity Remaining	Authorized Signature

Disposition of Unused Drug

Date	Disposition Method / Notes	Authorized Signature

PATIENT NARCOTIC'S LOG

Page Start Date	From Page #	To Page #

Patient Information

Last Name	First Name	Middle Name/Init.	Room # Bed#

Medication Name	Rx #	Prescribing Physician

☐ Oral ☐ Hypo ☐ Rectal

Initial Quantity Rec'd	Date Received	Pharmacy

Dosage / Directions

#	Date	Time	On Hand	Given	Rem-aining	From RX	Nurse Signature	Verified By Signature	Date	Time	Notes
1											
2											
3											
4											
5											
6											
7											
8											
9											
10											
11											
12											
13											
14											
15											
16											

(Quantity spans On Hand / Given / Remaining / From RX)

Drug Depleted?	Date	Time	Signature

Date	Medication Quantity Remaining	Authorized Signature

Disposition of Unused Drug

Date	Disposition Method / Notes	Authorized Signature

PATIENT NARCOTIC'S LOG

Page Start Date	From Page # To Page #

Patient Information

Last Name	First Name	Middle Name/Init.	Room #	Bed#

Medication Name	Rx #	Prescribing Physician

☐ Oral	☐ Hypo	☐ Rectal	Initial Quantity Rec'd	Date Received	Pharmacy

Dosage / Directions

#	Date	Time	On Hand	Quantity Given	Quantity Rem-aining	From RX	Nurse Signature	Verified By Signature	Date	Time	Notes
1											
2											
3											
4											
5											
6											
7											
8											
9											
10											
11											
12											
13											
14											
15											
16											

Drug Depleted?	Date	Time	Signature

Date	Medication Quantity Remaining	Authorized Signature

Disposition of Unused Drug

Date	Disposition Method / Notes	Authorized Signature

PATIENT NARCOTIC'S LOG

Page Start Date	From Page #	To Page #

Patient Information

Last Name	First Name	Middle Name/Init.	Room #	Bed#

Medication Name	Rx #	Prescribing Physician

☐ Oral	☐ Hypo	☐ Rectal	Initial Quantity Rec'd	Date Received	Pharmacy

Dosage / Directions

#	Date	Time	Quantity On Hand	Quantity Given	Quantity Rem-aining	From RX	Nurse Signature	Verified By Signature	Date	Time	Notes
1											
2											
3											
4											
5											
6											
7											
8											
9											
10											
11											
12											
13											
14											
15											
16											

Drug Depleted?	Date	Time	Signature

Date	Medication Quantity Remaining	Authorized Signature

Disposition of Unused Drug

Date	Disposition Method / Notes	Authorized Signature

PATIENT NARCOTIC'S LOG

Page Start Date	From Page #	To Page #

Patient Information

Last Name	First Name	Middle Name/Init.	Room #	Bed#

Medication Name	Rx #	Prescribing Physician

☐ Oral	☐ Hypo	☐ Rectal	Initial Quantity Rec'd	Date Received	Pharmacy

Dosage / Directions

#	Date	Time	On Hand	Quantity Given	Quantity Rem-aining	From RX	Nurse Signature	Verified By Signature	Date	Time	Notes
1											
2											
3											
4											
5											
6											
7											
8											
9											
10											
11											
12											
13											
14											
15											
16											

Drug Depleted?	Date	Time	Signature

Date	Medication Quantity Remaining	Authorized Signature

Disposition of Unused Drug

Date	Disposition Method / Notes	Authorized Signature

PATIENT NARCOTIC'S LOG

Page Start Date	From Page #	To Page #

Patient Information

Last Name	First Name	Middle Name/Init.	Room #	Bed#

Medication Name	Rx #	Prescribing Physician

☐ Oral	☐ Hypo	☐ Rectal	Initial Quantity Rec'd	Date Received	Pharmacy

Dosage / Directions

#	Date	Time	On Hand	Quantity Given	Quantity Rem-aining	From RX	Nurse Signature	Verified By Signature	Date	Time	Notes
1											
2											
3											
4											
5											
6											
7											
8											
9											
10											
11											
12											
13											
14											
15											
16											

Drug Depleted?	Date	Time	Signature

Date	Medication Quantity Remaining	Authorized Signature

Disposition of Unused Drug

Date	Disposition Method / Notes	Authorized Signature

PATIENT NARCOTIC'S LOG

Page Start Date	From Page #	To Page #

Patient Information

Last Name	First Name	Middle Name/Init.	Room #	Bed#

Medication Name	Rx #	Prescribing Physician

			Initial Quantity Rec'd	Date Received	Pharmacy
☐	☐	☐			
Oral	Hypo	Rectal			

Dosage / Directions

#	Date	Time	On Hand	Quantity Given	Quantity Rem-aining	From RX	Nurse Signature	Verified By Signature	Date	Time	Notes
1											
2											
3											
4											
5											
6											
7											
8											
9											
10											
11											
12											
13											
14											
15											
16											

Drug Depleted?	Date	Time	Signature

Date	Medication Quantity Remaining	Authorized Signature

Disposition of Unused Drug

Date	Disposition Method / Notes	Authorized Signature

PATIENT NARCOTIC'S LOG

Page Start Date	From Page #	To Page #

Patient Information

Last Name	First Name	Middle Name/Init.	Room #	Bed#

Medication Name	Rx #	Prescribing Physician

☐ Oral	☐ Hypo	☐ Rectal	Initial Quantity Rec'd	Date Received	Pharmacy

Dosage / Directions

#	Date	Time	On Hand	Quantity Given	Quantity Rem-aining	From RX	Nurse Signature	Verified By Signature	Date	Time	Notes
1											
2											
3											
4											
5											
6											
7											
8											
9											
10											
11											
12											
13											
14											
15											
16											

Drug Depleted?	Date	Time	Signature

Date	Medication Quantity Remaining	Authorized Signature

Disposition of Unused Drug

Date	Disposition Method / Notes	Authorized Signature

PATIENT NARCOTIC'S LOG

Patient Information

Last Name	First Name	Middle Name/Init.	Room #	Bed#

Medication Name	Rx #	Prescribing Physician

☐ Oral ☐ Hypo ☐ Rectal

Initial Quantity Rec'd	Date Received	Pharmacy

Dosage / Directions

#	Date	Time	Quantity On Hand	Quantity Given	Quantity Rem-aining	From RX	Nurse Signature	Verified By Signature	Date	Time	Notes
1											
2											
3											
4											
5											
6											
7											
8											
9											
10											
11											
12											
13											
14											
15											
16											

Drug Depleted?	Date	Time	Signature

Date	Medication Quantity Remaining	Authorized Signature

Disposition of Unused Drug

Date	Disposition Method / Notes	Authorized Signature

PATIENT NARCOTIC'S LOG

Page Start Date	From Page #	To Page #

Patient Information

Last Name	First Name

Middle Name/Init. | Room # | Bed#

Medication Name	Rx #	Prescribing Physician

☐ Oral	☐ Hypo	☐ Rectal	Initial Quantity Rec'd	Date Received	Pharmacy

Dosage / Directions

#	Date	Time	Quantity On Hand	Quantity Given	Quantity Rem-aining	Quantity From RX	Nurse Signature	Verified By Signature	Date	Time	Notes
1											
2											
3											
4											
5											
6											
7											
8											
9											
10											
11											
12											
13											
14											
15											
16											

Drug Depleted?	Date	Time	Signature

Date	Medication Quantity Remaining	Authorized Signature

Disposition of Unused Drug

Date	Disposition Method / Notes	Authorized Signature

PATIENT NARCOTIC'S LOG

Page Start Date	From Page #	To Page #

Patient Information

Last Name	First Name	Middle Name/Init.	Room #	Bed#

Medication Name	Rx #	Prescribing Physician

☐ Oral ☐ Hypo ☐ Rectal	Initial Quantity Rec'd	Date Received	Pharmacy

Dosage / Directions

#	Date	Time	On Hand	Quantity Given	Quantity Rem- aining	From RX	Nurse Signature	Verified By Signature	Date	Time	Notes
1											
2											
3											
4											
5											
6											
7											
8											
9											
10											
11											
12											
13											
14											
15											
16											

Drug Depleted?	Date	Time	Signature

Date	Medication Quantity Remaining	Authorized Signature

Disposition of Unused Drug

Date	Disposition Method / Notes	Authorized Signature

PATIENT NARCOTIC'S LOG

Page Start Date	From Page #	To Page #

Patient Information

Last Name	First Name	Middle Name/Init.	Room #　Bed#

Medication Name	Rx #	Prescribing Physician

☐ Oral	☐ Hypo	☐ Rectal	Initial Quantity Rec'd	Date Received	Pharmacy

Dosage / Directions

#	Date	Time	On Hand	Quantity Given	Quantity Rem-aining	From RX	Nurse Signature	Verified By Signature	Date	Time	Notes
1											
2											
3											
4											
5											
6											
7											
8											
9											
10											
11											
12											
13											
14											
15											
16											

Drug Depleted?	Date	Time	Signature

Date	Medication Quantity Remaining	Authorized Signature

Disposition of Unused Drug

Date	Disposition Method / Notes	Authorized Signature

PATIENT NARCOTIC'S LOG

Page Start Date	From Page #	To Page #

Patient Information

Last Name	First Name	Middle Name/Init. Room #	Bed#

Medication Name	Rx #	Prescribing Physician

☐ ☐ ☐
Oral Hypo Rectal

Initial Quantity Rec'd	Date Received	Pharmacy

Dosage / Directions

#	Date	Time	Quantity On Hand	Given	Rem-aining	From RX	Nurse Signature	Verified By Signature	Date	Time	Notes
1											
2											
3											
4											
5											
6											
7											
8											
9											
10											
11											
12											
13											
14											
15											
16											

Drug Depleted?	Date	Time	Signature

Date	Medication Quantity Remaining	Authorized Signature

Disposition of Unused Drug

Date	Disposition Method / Notes	Authorized Signature

PATIENT NARCOTIC'S LOG

Page Start Date	From Page #	To Page #

Patient Information

Last Name	First Name	Middle Name/Init.	Room #	Bed#

Medication Name	Rx #	Prescribing Physician

☐ Oral	☐ Hypo	☐ Rectal	Initial Quantity Rec'd	Date Received	Pharmacy

Dosage / Directions

#	Date	Time	On Hand	Quantity Given	Rem-aining	From RX	Nurse Signature	Verified By Signature	Date	Time	Notes
1											
2											
3											
4											
5											
6											
7											
8											
9											
10											
11											
12											
13											
14											
15											
16											

Drug Depleted?	Date	Time	Signature

Date	Medication Quantity Remaining	Authorized Signature

Disposition of Unused Drug

Date	Disposition Method / Notes	Authorized Signature

PATIENT NARCOTIC'S LOG

Page Start Date	From Page #	To Page #

Patient Information

Last Name	First Name	Middle Name/Init.	Room #	Bed#

Medication Name	Rx #	Prescribing Physician

☐ Oral ☐ Hypo ☐ Rectal	Initial Quantity Rec'd	Date Received	Pharmacy

Dosage / Directions

#	Date	Time	On Hand	Quantity Given	Quantity Rem-aining	From RX	Nurse Signature	Verified By Signature	Date	Time	Notes
1											
2											
3											
4											
5											
6											
7											
8											
9											
10											
11											
12											
13											
14											
15											
16											

Drug Depleted?	Date	Time	Signature

Date	Medication Quantity Remaining	Authorized Signature

Disposition of Unused Drug

Date	Disposition Method / Notes	Authorized Signature

PATIENT NARCOTIC'S LOG

Page Start Date	From Page #	To Page #

Patient Information

Last Name	First Name	Middle Name/Init.	Room #	Bed#

Medication Name	Rx #	Prescribing Physician

☐ Oral ☐ Hypo ☐ Rectal

Initial Quantity Rec'd	Date Received	Pharmacy

Dosage / Directions

#	Date	Time	Quantity On Hand	Quantity Given	Quantity Rem-aining	From RX	Nurse Signature	Verified By Signature	Date	Time	Notes
1											
2											
3											
4											
5											
6											
7											
8											
9											
10											
11											
12											
13											
14											
15											
16											

Drug Depleted?	Date	Time	Signature

Date	Medication Quantity Remaining	Authorized Signature

Disposition of Unused Drug

Date	Disposition Method / Notes	Authorized Signature

PATIENT NARCOTIC'S LOG

	Page Start Date	From Page #	To Page #

Patient Information

Last Name	First Name	Middle Name/Init.	Room #	Bed#

Medication Name	Rx #	Prescribing Physician

Oral ☐ Hypo ☐ Rectal ☐	Initial Quantity Rec'd	Date Received	Pharmacy

Dosage / Directions

#	Date	Time	On Hand	Quantity Given	Quantity Rem-aining	From RX	Nurse Signature	Verified By Signature	Date	Time	Notes
1											
2											
3											
4											
5											
6											
7											
8											
9											
10											
11											
12											
13											
14											
15											
16											

Drug Depleted?	Date	Time	Signature

Date	Medication Quantity Remaining	Authorized Signature

Disposition of Unused Drug

Date	Disposition Method / Notes	Authorized Signature

PATIENT NARCOTIC'S LOG

Page Start Date	From Page #	To Page #

Patient Information

Last Name	First Name	Middle Name/Init.	Room #	Bed#

Medication Name	Rx #	Prescribing Physician

☐ Oral	☐ Hypo	☐ Rectal	Initial Quantity Rec'd	Date Received	Pharmacy

Dosage / Directions

#	Date	Time	Quantity On Hand	Quantity Given	Quantity Rem-aining	Quantity From RX	Nurse Signature	Verified By Signature	Date	Time	Notes
1											
2											
3											
4											
5											
6											
7											
8											
9											
10											
11											
12											
13											
14											
15											
16											

Drug Depleted?		Date	Time	Signature

Date	Medication Quantity Remaining	Authorized Signature

Disposition of Unused Drug

Date	Disposition Method / Notes	Authorized Signature

PATIENT NARCOTIC'S LOG

Page Start Date	From Page #	To Page #

Patient Information

Last Name	First Name	Middle Name/Init.	Room #	Bed#

Medication Name	Rx #	Prescribing Physician

			Initial Quantity Rec'd	Date Received	Pharmacy
☐	☐	☐			
Oral	Hypo	Rectal			

Dosage / Directions

#	Date	Time	On Hand	Quantity Given	Quantity Rem-aining	From RX	Nurse Signature	Verified By Signature	Date	Time	Notes
1											
2											
3											
4											
5											
6											
7											
8											
9											
10											
11											
12											
13											
14											
15											
16											

Drug Depleted?	Date	Time	Signature

Date	Medication Quantity Remaining	Authorized Signature

Disposition of Unused Drug

Date	Disposition Method / Notes	Authorized Signature

PATIENT NARCOTIC'S LOG

Page Start Date	From Page #	To Page #

Patient Information

Last Name	First Name	Middle Name/Init.	Room #	Bed#

Medication Name	Rx #	Prescribing Physician

			Initial Quantity Rec'd	Date Received	Pharmacy
☐ Oral	☐ Hypo	☐ Rectal			

Dosage / Directions

#	Date	Time	On Hand	Quantity Given	Quantity Rem-aining	From RX	Nurse Signature	Verified By Signature	Date	Time	Notes
1											
2											
3											
4											
5											
6											
7											
8											
9											
10											
11											
12											
13											
14											
15											
16											

Drug Depleted?	Date	Time	Signature

Date	Medication Quantity Remaining	Authorized Signature

Disposition of Unused Drug

Date	Disposition Method / Notes	Authorized Signature

PATIENT NARCOTIC'S LOG

Page Start Date	From Page #	To Page #

Patient Information

Last Name	First Name	Middle Name/Init.	Room #	Bed#

Medication Name	Rx #	Prescribing Physician

☐	☐	☐	Initial Quantity Rec'd	Date Received	Pharmacy
Oral	Hypo	Rectal			

Dosage / Directions

#	Date	Time	Quantity On Hand	Quantity Given	Quantity Rem-aining	Quantity From RX	Nurse Signature	Verified By Signature	Date	Time	Notes
1											
2											
3											
4											
5											
6											
7											
8											
9											
10											
11											
12											
13											
14											
15											
16											

Drug Depleted?	Date	Time	Signature

Date	Medication Quantity Remaining	Authorized Signature

Disposition of Unused Drug

Date	Disposition Method / Notes	Authorized Signature

PATIENT NARCOTIC'S LOG

	Page Start Date	From Page #	To Page #

Patient Information

Last Name	First Name	Middle Name/Init.	Room #	Bed#

Medication Name	Rx #	Prescribing Physician

☐ Oral	☐ Hypo	☐ Rectal	Initial Quantity Rec'd	Date Received	Pharmacy

Dosage / Directions

#	Date	Time	On Hand	Quantity Given	Quantity Rem-aining	From RX	Nurse Signature	Verified By Signature	Date	Time	Notes
1											
2											
3											
4											
5											
6											
7											
8											
9											
10											
11											
12											
13											
14											
15											
16											

Drug Depleted?	Date	Time	Signature

Date	Medication Quantity Remaining	Authorized Signature

Disposition of Unused Drug

Date	Disposition Method / Notes	Authorized Signature

PATIENT NARCOTIC'S LOG

<table>
<tr><td>Page Start Date</td><td>From Page #</td><td>To Page #</td></tr>
</table>

Patient Information

Last Name	First Name	Middle Name/Init.	Room #	Bed#

Medication Name	Rx #	Prescribing Physician

☐ Oral	☐ Hypo	☐ Rectal	Initial Quantity Rec'd	Date Received	Pharmacy

Dosage / Directions

#	Date	Time	On Hand	Quantity Given	Quantity Rem-aining	From RX	Nurse Signature	Verified By Signature	Date	Time	Notes
1											
2											
3											
4											
5											
6											
7											
8											
9											
10											
11											
12											
13											
14											
15											
16											

Drug Depleted?	Date	Time	Signature

Date	Medication Quantity Remaining	Authorized Signature

Disposition of Unused Drug

Date	Disposition Method / Notes	Authorized Signature

PATIENT NARCOTIC'S LOG

Page Start Date	From Page #	To Page #

Patient Information

Last Name	First Name	Middle Name/Init.	Room #	Bed#

Medication Name	Rx #	Prescribing Physician

☐ Oral	☐ Hypo	☐ Rectal	Initial Quantity Rec'd	Date Received	Pharmacy

Dosage / Directions

#	Date	Time	Quantity On Hand	Quantity Given	Quantity Rem-aining	Quantity From RX	Nurse Signature	Verified By Signature	Date	Time	Notes
1											
2											
3											
4											
5											
6											
7											
8											
9											
10											
11											
12											
13											
14											
15											
16											

Drug Depleted?	Date	Time	Signature

Date	Medication Quantity Remaining	Authorized Signature

Disposition of Unused Drug		

Date	Disposition Method / Notes	Authorized Signature

PATIENT NARCOTIC'S LOG

Page Start Date	From Page #	To Page #

Patient Information

Last Name	First Name	Middle Name/Init.	Room #	Bed#

Medication Name	Rx #	Prescribing Physician

☐ Oral	☐ Hypo	☐ Rectal	Initial Quantity Rec'd	Date Received	Pharmacy

Dosage / Directions

#	Date	Time	Quantity On Hand	Given	Rem-aining	From RX	Nurse Signature	Verified By Signature	Date	Time	Notes
1											
2											
3											
4											
5											
6											
7											
8											
9											
10											
11											
12											
13											
14											
15											
16											

Drug Depleted?	Date	Time	Signature

Date	Medication Quantity Remaining	Authorized Signature

Disposition of Unused Drug

Date	Disposition Method / Notes	Authorized Signature

PATIENT NARCOTIC'S LOG

Page Start Date	From Page #	To Page #

Patient Information

Last Name	First Name	Middle Name/Init.	Room #	Bed#

Medication Name	Rx #	Prescribing Physician

☐ Oral	☐ Hypo	☐ Rectal	Initial Quantity Rec'd	Date Received	Pharmacy

Dosage / Directions

#	Date	Time	On Hand	Given	Rem-aining	From RX	Nurse Signature	Verified By Signature	Date	Time	Notes
1											
2											
3											
4											
5											
6											
7											
8											
9											
10											
11											
12											
13											
14											
15											
16											

Drug Depleted?	Date	Time	Signature

Date	Medication Quantity Remaining	Authorized Signature

Disposition of Unused Drug

Date	Disposition Method / Notes	Authorized Signature

PATIENT NARCOTIC'S LOG

Page Start Date	From Page #	To Page #

Patient Information

Last Name	First Name	Middle Name/Init.	Room # Bed#

Medication Name	Rx #	Prescribing Physician

☐ Oral	☐ Hypo	☐ Rectal	Initial Quantity Rec'd	Date Received	Pharmacy

Dosage / Directions

#	Date	Time	On Hand	Given	Quantity Rem-aining	From RX	Nurse Signature	Verified By Signature	Date	Time	Notes
1											
2											
3											
4											
5											
6											
7											
8											
9											
10											
11											
12											
13											
14											
15											
16											

Drug Depleted?	Date	Time	Signature

Date	Medication Quantity Remaining	Authorized Signature

Disposition of Unused Drug

Date	Disposition Method / Notes	Authorized Signature

PATIENT NARCOTIC'S LOG

Patient Information

Last Name	First Name	Middle Name/Init.	Room #	Bed#

Medication Name	Rx #	Prescribing Physician

☐	☐	☐	Initial Quantity Rec'd	Date Received	Pharmacy
Oral	Hypo	Rectal			

Dosage / Directions

#	Date	Time	On Hand	Given	Rem-aining	From RX	Nurse Signature	Verified By Signature	Date	Time	Notes
1											
2											
3											
4											
5											
6											
7											
8											
9											
10											
11											
12											
13											
14											
15											
16											

(Quantity spans the On Hand, Given, Rem-aining, From RX columns)

Drug Depleted?	Date	Time	Signature

Date	Medication Quantity Remaining	Authorized Signature

Disposition of Unused Drug

Date	Disposition Method / Notes	Authorized Signature

PATIENT NARCOTIC'S LOG

Page Start Date	From Page #	To Page #

Patient Information

Last Name	First Name	Middle Name/Init.	Room #	Bed#

Medication Name	Rx #	Prescribing Physician

☐	☐	☐	Initial Quantity Rec'd	Date Received	Pharmacy
Oral	Hypo	Rectal			

Dosage / Directions

#	Date	Time	On Hand	Given	Quantity Rem-aining	From RX	Nurse Signature	Verified By Signature	Date	Time	Notes
1											
2											
3											
4											
5											
6											
7											
8											
9											
10											
11											
12											
13											
14											
15											
16											

Drug Depleted?	Date	Time	Signature

Date	Medication Quantity Remaining	Authorized Signature

Disposition of Unused Drug

Date	Disposition Method / Notes	Authorized Signature

PATIENT NARCOTIC'S LOG

Page Start Date	From Page #	To Page #

Patient Information

Last Name	First Name	Middle Name/Init.	Room #	Bed#

Medication Name	Rx #	Prescribing Physician

☐ Oral	☐ Hypo	☐ Rectal	Initial Quantity Rec'd	Date Received	Pharmacy

Dosage / Directions

#	Date	Time	Quantity On Hand	Quantity Given	Quantity Rem-aining	Quantity From RX	Nurse Signature	Verified By Signature	Date	Time	Notes
1											
2											
3											
4											
5											
6											
7											
8											
9											
10											
11											
12											
13											
14											
15											
16											

Drug Depleted?	Date	Time	Signature

Date	Medication Quantity Remaining	Authorized Signature

Disposition of Unused Drug

Date	Disposition Method / Notes	Authorized Signature

PATIENT NARCOTIC'S LOG

Page Start Date	From Page #	To Page #

Patient Information

Last Name	First Name	Middle Name/Init.	Room #	Bed#

Medication Name	Rx #	Prescribing Physician

☐ Oral	☐ Hypo	☐ Rectal	Initial Quantity Rec'd	Date Received	Pharmacy

Dosage / Directions

#	Date	Time	Quantity On Hand	Quantity Given	Quantity Rem-aining	Quantity From RX	Nurse Signature	Verified By Signature	Date	Time	Notes
1											
2											
3											
4											
5											
6											
7											
8											
9											
10											
11											
12											
13											
14											
15											
16											

Drug Depleted?	Date	Time	Signature

Date	Medication Quantity Remaining	Authorized Signature

Disposition of Unused Drug		

Date	Disposition Method / Notes	Authorized Signature

PATIENT NARCOTIC'S LOG

Page Start Date	From Page #	To Page #

Patient Information

Last Name	First Name	Middle Name/Init.	Room #	Bed#

Medication Name	Rx #	Prescribing Physician

☐ Oral	☐ Hypo	☐ Rectal	Initial Quantity Rec'd	Date Received	Pharmacy

Dosage / Directions

#	Date	Time	On Hand	Quantity Given	Quantity Rem-aining	From RX	Nurse Signature	Verified By Signature	Date	Time	Notes
1											
2											
3											
4											
5											
6											
7											
8											
9											
10											
11											
12											
13											
14											
15											
16											

Drug Depleted?	Date	Time	Signature

Date	Medication Quantity Remaining	Authorized Signature

Disposition of Unused Drug

Date	Disposition Method / Notes	Authorized Signature

PATIENT NARCOTIC'S LOG

Patient Information

Last Name	First Name	Middle Name/Init.	Room #	Bed#

Medication Name | Rx # | Prescribing Physician

☐ Oral	☐ Hypo	☐ Rectal	Initial Quantity Rec'd	Date Received	Pharmacy

Dosage / Directions

#	Date	Time	Quantity				Nurse Signature	Verified By Signature	Date	Time	Notes
			On Hand	Given	Rem-aining	From RX					
1											
2											
3											
4											
5											
6											
7											
8											
9											
10											
11											
12											
13											
14											
15											
16											

Drug Depleted?	Date	Time	Signature

Date	Medication Quantity Remaining	Authorized Signature

Disposition of Unused Drug

Date	Disposition Method / Notes	Authorized Signature

PATIENT NARCOTIC'S LOG

Page Start Date	From Page #	To Page #

Patient Information

Last Name	First Name	Middle Name/Init.	Room # Bed#

Medication Name	Rx #	Prescribing Physician

			Initial Quantity Rec'd	Date Received	Pharmacy
☐ Oral	☐ Hypo	☐ Rectal			

Dosage / Directions

#	Date	Time	Quantity On Hand	Quantity Given	Quantity Rem-aining	Quantity From RX	Nurse Signature	Verified By Signature	Date	Time	Notes
1											
2											
3											
4											
5											
6											
7											
8											
9											
10											
11											
12											
13											
14											
15											
16											

Drug Depleted?	Date	Time	Signature

Date	Medication Quantity Remaining	Authorized Signature

Disposition of Unused Drug		

Date	Disposition Method / Notes	Authorized Signature

PATIENT NARCOTIC'S LOG

Page Start Date	From Page #	To Page #

Patient Information

Last Name	First Name	Middle Name/Init.	Room #	Bed#

Medication Name	Rx #	Prescribing Physician

			Initial Quantity Rec'd	Date Received	Pharmacy
☐ Oral	☐ Hypo	☐ Rectal			

Dosage / Directions

#	Date	Time	On Hand	Quantity Given	Quantity Rem-aining	From RX	Nurse Signature	Verified By Signature	Date	Time	Notes
1											
2											
3											
4											
5											
6											
7											
8											
9											
10											
11											
12											
13											
14											
15											
16											

Drug Depleted?	Date	Time	Signature

Date	Medication Quantity Remaining	Authorized Signature

Disposition of Unused Drug

Date	Disposition Method / Notes	Authorized Signature

PATIENT NARCOTIC'S LOG

Page Start Date	From Page #	To Page #

Patient Information

Last Name	First Name	Middle Name/Init.	Room #	Bed#

Medication Name	Rx #	Prescribing Physician

☐ Oral	☐ Hypo	☐ Rectal	Initial Quantity Rec'd	Date Received	Pharmacy

Dosage / Directions

#	Date	Time	On Hand	Quantity Given	Rem-aining	From RX	Nurse Signature	Verified By Signature	Date	Time	Notes
1											
2											
3											
4											
5											
6											
7											
8											
9											
10											
11											
12											
13											
14											
15											
16											

Drug Depleted?	Date	Time	Signature

Date	Medication Quantity Remaining	Authorized Signature

Disposition of Unused Drug

Date	Disposition Method / Notes	Authorized Signature

PATIENT NARCOTIC'S LOG

Page Start Date	From Page #	To Page #

Patient Information

Last Name	First Name	Middle Name/Init.	Room #	Bed#

Medication Name	Rx #	Prescribing Physician

☐	☐	☐	Initial Quantity Rec'd	Date Received	Pharmacy
Oral	Hypo	Rectal			

Dosage / Directions

#	Date	Time	Quantity On Hand	Given	Rem-aining	From RX	Nurse Signature	Verified By Signature	Date	Time	Notes
1											
2											
3											
4											
5											
6											
7											
8											
9											
10											
11											
12											
13											
14											
15											
16											

Drug Depleted?	Date	Time	Signature

Date	Medication Quantity Remaining	Authorized Signature

Disposition of Unused Drug

Date	Disposition Method / Notes	Authorized Signature

PATIENT NARCOTIC'S LOG

Page Start Date	From Page #	To Page #

Patient Information

Last Name	First Name	Middle Name/Init. Room #	Bed#

Medication Name	Rx #	Prescribing Physician

			Initial Quantity Rec'd	Date Received	Pharmacy
☐ Oral	☐ Hypo	☐ Rectal			

Dosage / Directions

#	Date	Time	Quantity On Hand	Quantity Given	Quantity Rem-aining	From RX	Nurse Signature	Verified By Signature	Date	Time	Notes
1											
2											
3											
4											
5											
6											
7											
8											
9											
10											
11											
12											
13											
14											
15											
16											

Drug Depleted?	Date	Time	Signature

Date	Medication Quantity Remaining	Authorized Signature

Disposition of Unused Drug

Date	Disposition Method / Notes	Authorized Signature

PATIENT NARCOTIC'S LOG

	Page Start Date	From Page #	To Page #

Patient Information

Last Name	First Name	Middle Name/Init.	Room #	Bed#

Medication Name	Rx #	Prescribing Physician

☐ Oral	☐ Hypo	☐ Rectal	Initial Quantity Rec'd	Date Received	Pharmacy

Dosage / Directions

#	Date	Time	On Hand	Given	Rem-aining	From RX	Nurse Signature	Verified By Signature	Date	Time	Notes
1											
2											
3											
4											
5											
6											
7											
8											
9											
10											
11											
12											
13											
14											
15											
16											

Quantity (spanning On Hand, Given, Rem-aining, From RX)

Drug Depleted?	Date	Time	Signature

Date	Medication Quantity Remaining	Authorized Signature

Disposition of Unused Drug

Date	Disposition Method / Notes	Authorized Signature

PATIENT NARCOTIC'S LOG

Page Start Date	From Page #	To Page #

Patient Information

Last Name	First Name	Middle Name/Init.	Room #	Bed#

Medication Name	Rx #	Prescribing Physician

			Initial Quantity Rec'd	Date Received	Pharmacy
☐ Oral	☐ Hypo	☐ Rectal			

Dosage / Directions

#	Date	Time	On Hand	Quantity Given	Rem-aining	From RX	Nurse Signature	Verified By Signature	Date	Time	Notes
1											
2											
3											
4											
5											
6											
7											
8											
9											
10											
11											
12											
13											
14											
15											
16											

Drug Depleted?	Date	Time	Signature

Date	Medication Quantity Remaining	Authorized Signature

Disposition of Unused Drug

Date	Disposition Method / Notes	Authorized Signature

PATIENT NARCOTIC'S LOG

Page Start Date	From Page #	To Page #

Patient Information

Last Name	First Name	Middle Name/Init.	Room #	Bed#

Medication Name	Rx #	Prescribing Physician

☐ Oral	☐ Hypo	☐ Rectal	Initial Quantity Rec'd	Date Received	Pharmacy

Dosage / Directions

#	Date	Time	On Hand	Given	Remaining	From RX	Nurse Signature	Verified By Signature	Date	Time	Notes
1											
2											
3											
4											
5											
6											
7											
8											
9											
10											
11											
12											
13											
14											
15											
16											

Drug Depleted?	Date	Time	Signature

Date	Medication Quantity Remaining	Authorized Signature

Disposition of Unused Drug

Date	Disposition Method / Notes	Authorized Signature

PATIENT NARCOTIC'S LOG

Page Start Date	From Page #	To Page #

Patient Information

Last Name	First Name	Middle Name/Init.	Room #	Bed#

Medication Name	Rx #	Prescribing Physician

	Oral	Hypo	Rectal	Initial Quantity Rec'd	Date Received	Pharmacy
☐	☐	☐				

Dosage / Directions

#	Date	Time	On Hand	Given	Remaining	From RX	Nurse Signature	Verified By Signature	Date	Time	Notes
1											
2											
3											
4											
5											
6											
7											
8											
9											
10											
11											
12											
13											
14											
15											
16											

Drug Depleted?	Date	Time	Signature

Date	Medication Quantity Remaining	Authorized Signature

Disposition of Unused Drug

Date	Disposition Method / Notes	Authorized Signature

PATIENT NARCOTIC'S LOG

	Page Start Date	From Page #	To Page #

Patient Information

Last Name		First Name		Middle Name/Init.	Room #	Bed#

Medication Name	Rx #	Prescribing Physician

☐ Oral	☐ Hypo	☐ Rectal	Initial Quantity Rec'd	Date Received	Pharmacy

Dosage / Directions

#	Date	Time	Quantity On Hand	Given	Rem-aining	From RX	Nurse Signature	Verified By Signature	Date	Time	Notes
1											
2											
3											
4											
5											
6											
7											
8											
9											
10											
11											
12											
13											
14											
15											
16											

Drug Depleted?	Date	Time	Signature

Date	Medication Quantity Remaining	Authorized Signature

Disposition of Unused Drug		

Date	Disposition Method / Notes	Authorized Signature

PATIENT NARCOTIC'S LOG

Page Start Date	From Page #	To Page #

Patient Information

Last Name	First Name	Middle Name/Init.	Room #	Bed#

Medication Name	Rx #	Prescribing Physician

☐ Oral	☐ Hypo	☐ Rectal	Initial Quantity Rec'd	Date Received	Pharmacy

Dosage / Directions

#	Date	Time	On Hand	Quantity Given	Rem-aining	From RX	Nurse Signature	Verified By Signature	Date	Time	Notes
1											
2											
3											
4											
5											
6											
7											
8											
9											
10											
11											
12											
13											
14											
15											
16											

Drug Depleted?	Date	Time	Signature

Date	Medication Quantity Remaining	Authorized Signature

Disposition of Unused Drug

Date	Disposition Method / Notes	Authorized Signature

PATIENT NARCOTIC'S LOG

	Page Start Date	From Page #	To Page #

Patient Information

Last Name	First Name	Middle Name/Init.	Room #	Bed#

Medication Name	Rx #	Prescribing Physician

☐ Oral ☐ Hypo ☐ Rectal

Initial Quantity Rec'd	Date Received	Pharmacy

Dosage / Directions

#	Date	Time	On Hand	Quantity Given	Quantity Rem-aining	Quantity From RX	Nurse Signature	Verified By Signature	Date	Time	Notes
1											
2											
3											
4											
5											
6											
7											
8											
9											
10											
11											
12											
13											
14											
15											
16											

Drug Depleted?	Date	Time	Signature

Date	Medication Quantity Remaining	Authorized Signature

Disposition of Unused Drug

Date	Disposition Method / Notes	Authorized Signature

PATIENT NARCOTIC'S LOG

Page Start Date	From Page #	To Page #

Patient Information

Last Name	First Name	Middle Name/Init.	Room #	Bed#

Medication Name	Rx #	Prescribing Physician

☐ Oral	☐ Hypo	☐ Rectal	Initial Quantity Rec'd	Date Received	Pharmacy

Dosage / Directions

#	Date	Time	Quantity On Hand	Quantity Given	Quantity Rem-aining	Quantity From RX	Nurse Signature	Verified By Signature	Date	Time	Notes
1											
2											
3											
4											
5											
6											
7											
8											
9											
10											
11											
12											
13											
14											
15											
16											

Drug Depleted?	Date	Time	Signature

Date	Medication Quantity Remaining	Authorized Signature

Disposition of Unused Drug

Date	Disposition Method / Notes	Authorized Signature

PATIENT NARCOTIC'S LOG

Page Start Date	From Page #	To Page #

Patient Information

Last Name	First Name	Middle Name/Init.	Room #	Bed#

Medication Name	Rx #	Prescribing Physician

☐ Oral	☐ Hypo	☐ Rectal	Initial Quantity Rec'd	Date Received	Pharmacy

Dosage / Directions

#	Date	Time	On Hand	Quantity Given	Quantity Rem-aining	From RX	Nurse Signature	Verified By Signature	Date	Time	Notes
1											
2											
3											
4											
5											
6											
7											
8											
9											
10											
11											
12											
13											
14											
15											
16											

Drug Depleted?	Date	Time	Signature

Date	Medication Quantity Remaining	Authorized Signature

Disposition of Unused Drug

Date	Disposition Method / Notes	Authorized Signature

PATIENT NARCOTIC'S LOG

Page Start Date	From Page #	To Page #

Patient Information

Last Name	First Name	Middle Name/Init.	Room #	Bed#

Medication Name	Rx #	Prescribing Physician

☐ Oral	☐ Hypo	☐ Rectal	Initial Quantity Rec'd	Date Received	Pharmacy

Dosage / Directions

#	Date	Time	Quantity On Hand	Quantity Given	Quantity Rem-aining	Quantity From RX	Nurse Signature	Verified By Signature	Date	Time	Notes
1											
2											
3											
4											
5											
6											
7											
8											
9											
10											
11											
12											
13											
14											
15											
16											

Drug Depleted?	Date	Time	Signature

Date	Medication Quantity Remaining	Authorized Signature

Disposition of Unused Drug

Date	Disposition Method / Notes	Authorized Signature

PATIENT NARCOTIC'S LOG

Page Start Date	From Page #	To Page #

Patient Information

Last Name	First Name	Middle Name/Init.	Room #	Bed#

Medication Name	Rx #	Prescribing Physician

☐ Oral	☐ Hypo	☐ Rectal	Initial Quantity Rec'd	Date Received	Pharmacy

Dosage / Directions

#	Date	Time	Quantity On Hand	Quantity Given	Quantity Rem-aining	From RX	Nurse Signature	Verified By Signature	Date	Time	Notes
1											
2											
3											
4											
5											
6											
7											
8											
9											
10											
11											
12											
13											
14											
15											
16											

Drug Depleted?	Date	Time	Signature

Date	Medication Quantity Remaining	Authorized Signature

Disposition of Unused Drug

Date	Disposition Method / Notes	Authorized Signature

PATIENT NARCOTIC'S LOG

Page Start Date	From Page #	To Page #

Patient Information

Last Name	First Name	Middle Name/Init.	Room #	Bed#

Medication Name	Rx #	Prescribing Physician

☐	☐	☐	Initial Quantity Rec'd		Date Received	Pharmacy
Oral	Hypo	Rectal				

Dosage / Directions

#	Date	Time	Quantity On Hand	Quantity Given	Quantity Rem-aining	From RX	Nurse Signature	Verified By Signature	Date	Time	Notes
1											
2											
3											
4											
5											
6											
7											
8											
9											
10											
11											
12											
13											
14											
15											
16											

Drug Depleted?	Date	Time	Signature

Date	Medication Quantity Remaining	Authorized Signature

Disposition of Unused Drug

Date	Disposition Method / Notes	Authorized Signature

PATIENT NARCOTIC'S LOG

Page Start Date	From Page #	To Page #

Patient Information

Last Name	First Name	Middle Name/Init.	Room #	Bed#

Medication Name	Rx #	Prescribing Physician

☐ Oral	☐ Hypo	☐ Rectal	Initial Quantity Rec'd	Date Received	Pharmacy

Dosage / Directions

#	Date	Time	On Hand	Quantity Given	Quantity Rem-aining	From RX	Nurse Signature	Verified By Signature	Date	Time	Notes
1											
2											
3											
4											
5											
6											
7											
8											
9											
10											
11											
12											
13											
14											
15											
16											

Drug Depleted?	Date	Time	Signature

Date	Medication Quantity Remaining	Authorized Signature

Disposition of Unused Drug

Date	Disposition Method / Notes	Authorized Signature

PATIENT NARCOTIC'S LOG

Page Start Date	From Page #	To Page #

Patient Information

Last Name	First Name	Middle Name/Init.	Room #	Bed#

Medication Name	Rx #	Prescribing Physician

☐ Oral	☐ Hypo	☐ Rectal	Initial Quantity Rec'd	Date Received	Pharmacy

Dosage / Directions

#	Date	Time	On Hand	Quantity Given	Quantity Rem-aining	From RX	Nurse Signature	Verified By Signature	Date	Time	Notes
1											
2											
3											
4											
5											
6											
7											
8											
9											
10											
11											
12											
13											
14											
15											
16											

Drug Depleted?	Date	Time	Signature

Date	Medication Quantity Remaining	Authorized Signature

Disposition of Unused Drug

Date	Disposition Method / Notes	Authorized Signature

PATIENT NARCOTIC'S LOG

Page Start Date	From Page #	To Page #

Patient Information

Last Name	First Name	Middle Name/Init.	Room #	Bed#

Medication Name	Rx #	Prescribing Physician

☐ Oral	☐ Hypo	☐ Rectal	Initial Quantity Rec'd	Date Received	Pharmacy

Dosage / Directions

#	Date	Time	On Hand	Quantity Given	Rem-aining	From RX	Nurse Signature	Verified By Signature	Date	Time	Notes
1											
2											
3											
4											
5											
6											
7											
8											
9											
10											
11											
12											
13											
14											
15											
16											

Drug Depleted?	Date	Time	Signature

Date	Medication Quantity Remaining	Authorized Signature

Disposition of Unused Drug

Date	Disposition Method / Notes	Authorized Signature

PATIENT NARCOTIC'S LOG

Page Start Date	From Page #	To Page #

Patient Information

Last Name	First Name	Middle Name/Init.	Room #	Bed#

Medication Name	Rx #	Prescribing Physician

			Initial Quantity Rec'd	Date Received	Pharmacy
☐ Oral	☐ Hypo	☐ Rectal			

Dosage / Directions

#	Date	Time	On Hand	Quantity Given	Quantity Rem-aining	From RX	Nurse Signature	Verified By Signature	Date	Time	Notes
1											
2											
3											
4											
5											
6											
7											
8											
9											
10											
11											
12											
13											
14											
15											
16											

Drug Depleted?	Date	Time	Signature

Date	Medication Quantity Remaining	Authorized Signature

Disposition of Unused Drug

Date	Disposition Method / Notes	Authorized Signature

PATIENT NARCOTIC'S LOG

Page Start Date	From Page #	To Page #

Patient Information

Last Name	First Name	Middle Name/Init.	Room #	Bed#

Medication Name	Rx #	Prescribing Physician

☐ Oral	☐ Hypo	☐ Rectal	Initial Quantity Rec'd	Date Received	Pharmacy

Dosage / Directions

#	Date	Time	On Hand	Quantity Given	Quantity Rem-aining	From RX	Nurse Signature	Verified By Signature	Date	Time	Notes
1											
2											
3											
4											
5											
6											
7											
8											
9											
10											
11											
12											
13											
14											
15											
16											

Drug Depleted?	Date	Time	Signature

Date	Medication Quantity Remaining	Authorized Signature

Disposition of Unused Drug

Date	Disposition Method / Notes	Authorized Signature

PATIENT NARCOTIC'S LOG

Page Start Date	From Page #	To Page #

Patient Information

Last Name	First Name	Middle Name/Init.	Room #	Bed#

Medication Name	Rx #	Prescribing Physician

☐ Oral	☐ Hypo	☐ Rectal	Initial Quantity Rec'd	Date Received	Pharmacy

Dosage / Directions

#	Date	Time	Quantity On Hand	Quantity Given	Quantity Rem-aining	Quantity From RX	Nurse Signature	Verified By Signature	Date	Time	Notes
1											
2											
3											
4											
5											
6											
7											
8											
9											
10											
11											
12											
13											
14											
15											
16											

Drug Depleted?	Date	Time	Signature

Date	Medication Quantity Remaining	Authorized Signature

Disposition of Unused Drug		

Date	Disposition Method / Notes	Authorized Signature

PATIENT NARCOTIC'S LOG

Page Start Date	From Page #	To Page #

Patient Information

Last Name	First Name	Middle Name/Init.	Room #　Bed#

Medication Name	Rx #	Prescribing Physician

☐ Oral	☐ Hypo	☐ Rectal	Initial Quantity Rec'd	Date Received	Pharmacy

Dosage / Directions

#	Date	Time	On Hand	Given	Remaining	From RX	Nurse Signature	Verified By Signature	Date	Time	Notes
1											
2											
3											
4											
5											
6											
7											
8											
9											
10											
11											
12											
13											
14											
15											
16											

(Quantity columns: On Hand, Given, Remaining, From RX)

Drug Depleted?	Date	Time	Signature

Date	Medication Quantity Remaining	Authorized Signature

Disposition of Unused Drug		

Date	Disposition Method / Notes	Authorized Signature

PATIENT NARCOTIC'S LOG

Page Start Date	From Page #	To Page #

Patient Information

Last Name	First Name	Middle Name/Init.	Room #	Bed#

Medication Name	Rx #	Prescribing Physician

☐ Oral	☐ Hypo	☐ Rectal	Initial Quantity Rec'd	Date Received	Pharmacy

Dosage / Directions

#	Date	Time	On Hand	Quantity Given	Quantity Rem-aining	From RX	Nurse Signature	Verified By Signature	Date	Time	Notes
1											
2											
3											
4											
5											
6											
7											
8											
9											
10											
11											
12											
13											
14											
15											
16											

Drug Depleted?	Date	Time	Signature

Date	Medication Quantity Remaining	Authorized Signature

Disposition of Unused Drug

Date	Disposition Method / Notes	Authorized Signature

PATIENT NARCOTIC'S LOG

Page Start Date	From Page #	To Page #

Patient Information

Last Name	First Name	Middle Name/Init.	Room #	Bed#

Medication Name	Rx #	Prescribing Physician

☐ Oral	☐ Hypo	☐ Rectal	Initial Quantity Rec'd	Date Received	Pharmacy

Dosage / Directions

#	Date	Time	On Hand	Given	Rem-aining	From RX	Nurse Signature	Verified By Signature	Date	Time	Notes
				Quantity							
1											
2											
3											
4											
5											
6											
7											
8											
9											
10											
11											
12											
13											
14											
15											
16											

Drug Depleted?	Date	Time	Signature

Date	Medication Quantity Remaining	Authorized Signature

Disposition of Unused Drug

Date	Disposition Method / Notes	Authorized Signature

PATIENT NARCOTIC'S LOG

Page Start Date	From Page #	To Page #

Patient Information

Last Name	First Name	Middle Name/Init.	Room #	Bed#

Medication Name	Rx #	Prescribing Physician

☐ Oral	☐ Hypo	☐ Rectal	Initial Quantity Rec'd	Date Received	Pharmacy

Dosage / Directions

#	Date	Time	Quantity On Hand	Quantity Given	Quantity Rem-aining	Quantity From RX	Nurse Signature	Verified By Signature	Date	Time	Notes
1											
2											
3											
4											
5											
6											
7											
8											
9											
10											
11											
12											
13											
14											
15											
16											

Drug Depleted?	Date	Time	Signature

Date	Medication Quantity Remaining	Authorized Signature

Disposition of Unused Drug

Date	Disposition Method / Notes	Authorized Signature

PATIENT NARCOTIC'S LOG

Page Start Date	From Page #	To Page #

Patient Information

Last Name	First Name	Middle Name/Init.	Room #	Bed#

Medication Name	Rx #	Prescribing Physician

☐ Oral ☐ Hypo ☐ Rectal	Initial Quantity Rec'd	Date Received	Pharmacy

Dosage / Directions

#	Date	Time	Quantity On Hand	Quantity Given	Quantity Rem-aining	From RX	Nurse Signature	Verified By Signature	Date	Time	Notes
1											
2											
3											
4											
5											
6											
7											
8											
9											
10											
11											
12											
13											
14											
15											
16											

Drug Depleted?	Date	Time	Signature

Date	Medication Quantity Remaining	Authorized Signature

Disposition of Unused Drug

Date	Disposition Method / Notes	Authorized Signature

PATIENT NARCOTIC'S LOG

Page Start Date	From Page #	To Page #

Patient Information

Last Name	First Name	Middle Name/Init.	Room #	Bed#

Medication Name	Rx #	Prescribing Physician

☐ Oral ☐ Hypo ☐ Rectal

Initial Quantity Rec'd	Date Received	Pharmacy

Dosage / Directions

#	Date	Time	Quantity			Nurse Signature	Verified By Signature	Date	Time	Notes
			On Hand	Given	Rem-aining	From RX				
1											
2											
3											
4											
5											
6											
7											
8											
9											
10											
11											
12											
13											
14											
15											
16											

Drug Depleted?	Date	Time	Signature

Date	Medication Quantity Remaining	Authorized Signature

Disposition of Unused Drug

Date	Disposition Method / Notes	Authorized Signature

PATIENT NARCOTIC'S LOG

Patient Information

Last Name	First Name	Middle Name/Init.	Room #	Bed#

Medication Name	Rx #	Prescribing Physician

☐ Oral	☐ Hypo	☐ Rectal	Initial Quantity Rec'd	Date Received	Pharmacy

Dosage / Directions

#	Date	Time	On Hand	Quantity Given	Quantity Rem-aining	From RX	Nurse Signature	Verified By Signature	Date	Time	Notes
1											
2											
3											
4											
5											
6											
7											
8											
9											
10											
11											
12											
13											
14											
15											
16											

Drug Depleted?	Date	Time	Signature

Date	Medication Quantity Remaining	Authorized Signature

Disposition of Unused Drug

Date	Disposition Method / Notes	Authorized Signature

PATIENT NARCOTIC'S LOG

Page Start Date	From Page #	To Page #

Patient Information

Last Name	First Name	Middle Name/Init.	Room #	Bed#

Medication Name	Rx #	Prescribing Physician

☐ Oral	☐ Hypo	☐ Rectal	Initial Quantity Rec'd	Date Received	Pharmacy

Dosage / Directions

#	Date	Time	Quantity On Hand	Quantity Given	Quantity Rem-aining	Quantity From RX	Nurse Signature	Verified By Signature	Date	Time	Notes
1											
2											
3											
4											
5											
6											
7											
8											
9											
10											
11											
12											
13											
14											
15											
16											

Drug Depleted?	Date	Time	Signature

Date	Medication Quantity Remaining	Authorized Signature

Disposition of Unused Drug

Date	Disposition Method / Notes	Authorized Signature

PATIENT NARCOTIC'S LOG

Page Start Date	From Page #	To Page #

Patient Information

Last Name	First Name	Middle Name/Init.	Room #	Bed#

Medication Name	Rx #	Prescribing Physician

☐ Oral	☐ Hypo	☐ Rectal	Initial Quantity Rec'd	Date Received	Pharmacy

Dosage / Directions

#	Date	Time	On Hand	Quantity Given	Quantity Rem-aining	From RX	Nurse Signature	Verified By Signature	Date	Time	Notes
1											
2											
3											
4											
5											
6											
7											
8											
9											
10											
11											
12											
13											
14											
15											
16											

Drug Depleted?	Date	Time	Signature

Date	Medication Quantity Remaining	Authorized Signature

Disposition of Unused Drug

Date	Disposition Method / Notes	Authorized Signature

PATIENT NARCOTIC'S LOG

Page Start Date	From Page #	To Page #

Patient Information

Last Name	First Name	Middle Name/Init.	Room #	Bed#

Medication Name	Rx #	Prescribing Physician

☐ Oral	☐ Hypo	☐ Rectal	Initial Quantity Rec'd	Date Received	Pharmacy

Dosage / Directions

#	Date	Time	Quantity On Hand	Quantity Given	Quantity Rem-aining	Quantity From RX	Nurse Signature	Verified By Signature	Date	Time	Notes
1											
2											
3											
4											
5											
6											
7											
8											
9											
10											
11											
12											
13											
14											
15											
16											

Drug Depleted?		Date	Time	Signature

Date	Medication Quantity Remaining	Authorized Signature

Disposition of Unused Drug

Date	Disposition Method / Notes	Authorized Signature

PATIENT NARCOTIC'S LOG

Page Start Date	From Page #	To Page #

Patient Information

Last Name	First Name	Middle Name/Init.	Room #	Bed#

Medication Name	Rx #	Prescribing Physician

☐ Oral	☐ Hypo	☐ Rectal	Initial Quantity Rec'd	Date Received	Pharmacy

Dosage / Directions

#	Date	Time	On Hand	Given	Remaining	From RX	Nurse Signature	Verified By Signature	Date	Time	Notes
1											
2											
3											
4											
5											
6											
7											
8											
9											
10											
11											
12											
13											
14											
15											
16											

(Quantity spans: On Hand, Given, Remaining, From RX)

Drug Depleted?	Date	Time	Signature

Date	Medication Quantity Remaining	Authorized Signature

Disposition of Unused Drug

Date	Disposition Method / Notes	Authorized Signature

Patient Index

Page #	Patient Name	Drug Name / Rx #	Physician	Start Date	End Date
1					
2					
3					
4					
5					
6					
7					
8					
9					
10					
11					
12					
13					
14					
15					
16					
17					
18					
19					
20					
21					
22					
23					
24					
25					
26					
27					
28					
29					
30					
31					
32					
33					
34					
35					

Patient Index

Page #	Patient Name	Drug Name / Rx #	Physician	Start Date	End Date
36					
37					
38					
39					
40					
41					
42					
43					
44					
45					
46					
47					
48					
49					
50					
51					
52					
53					
54					
55					
56					
57					
58					
59					
60					
61					
62					
63					
64					
65					
66					
67					
68					
69					
70					

Patient Index

Page #	Patient Name	Drug Name / Rx #	Physician	Start Date	End Date
71					
72					
73					
74					
75					
76					
77					
78					
79					
80					
81					
82					
83					
84					
85					
86					
87					
88					
89					
90					
91					
92					
93					
94					
95					
96					
97					
98					
99					
100					
101					
102					
103					
104					
105					

Patient Index

Page #	Patient Name	Drug Name / Rx #	Physician	Start Date	End Date
106					
107					
108					
109					
110					
111					
112					
113					
114					
115					
116					
117					
118					
119					
120					
121					
122					
123					
124					
125					
126					
127					
128					
129					
130